Discover Secret Anti-Aging Juice & Tonic Recipes

"Unique Juices And Tonics That Create Beauty And Youth"

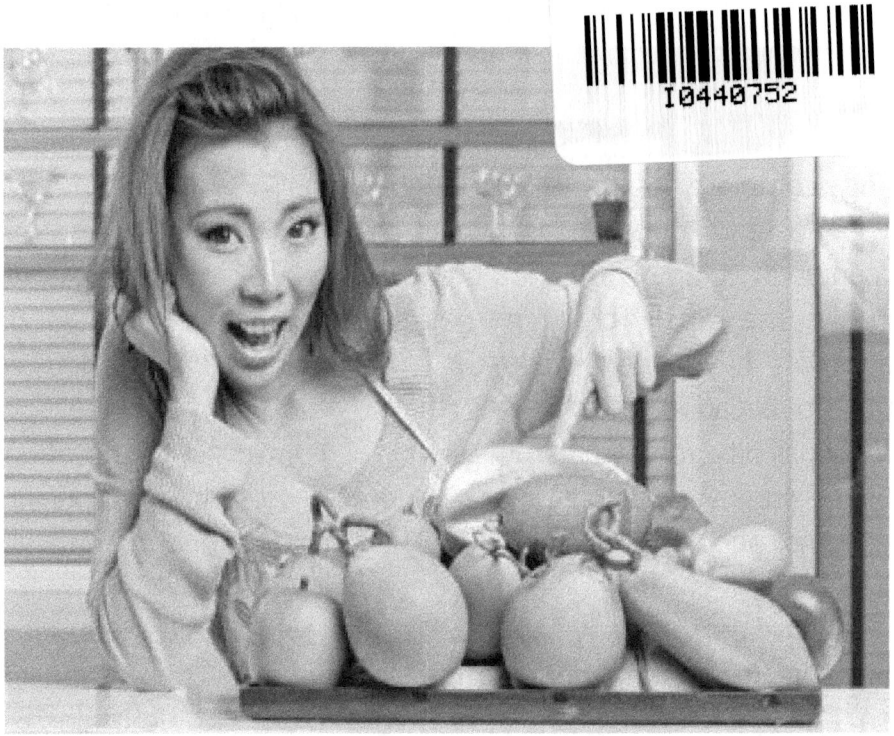

By Rudy Silva Silva, Natural Nutritionist

Discover Secret Anti-Aging Juice & Tonic Recipes © 2013 by Rudy S Silva, All Rights Reserved.

Disclaimer and Terms of Use:

All Rights Reserved.   No part of this publication may be reproduced in any form or by any means, including scanning, photocopying, or otherwise without prior written permission of the copyright holder.

The Author and Publisher have strived to be as accurate and complete as possible in the creation of this book, notwithstanding the fact that he does not warrant or represent at any time that the contents within are accurate due to the rapidly changing nature of the Internet. While all attempts have been made to verify information provided in this publication, the Author and Publisher assume no responsibility for errors, omissions, or contrary interpretation of the subject matter herein. Any perceived slights of specific persons, peoples, or organizations are unintentional.

All readers are advised to seek their own medical help.
The information here is for educational purposes and in no way is it medical advice or treatment. Ask your doctor before using any of the natural remedies listed here.

First Printing, 2013 printed in the United States of America

Table of Contents

1: Introduction To Anti-Aging Secrets

2: Why Juices Are Anti-Aging

3: The Anti-aging Power of Enzymes

4: How Fruit Minerals Burn Acid

5: Fruits to Eat And Drink To Preserve Youth

6: Fruit Juices That Create Youth & Health

7: The Power of Vegetable To Keep You, Young

8: What You Should Know About Vegetable Juices

9: The Cures From Vegetable Juice

10: Special Tonics That Block Aging & Promote Youth

11: Basic Principle Of Smoothies That Give Health

12: When To Drink Your Juices

13: Natural Body Cycle 2

14: Natural Body Cycle 3

15: Juice and Tonic Program

16: The Author And Other Resources

1: Introduction To Anti-Aging Secrets

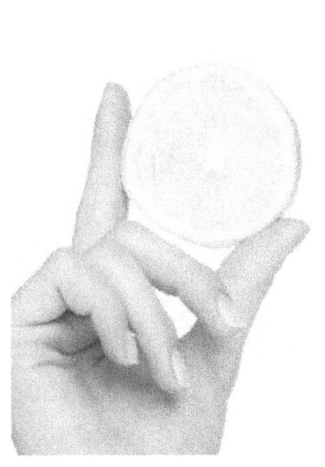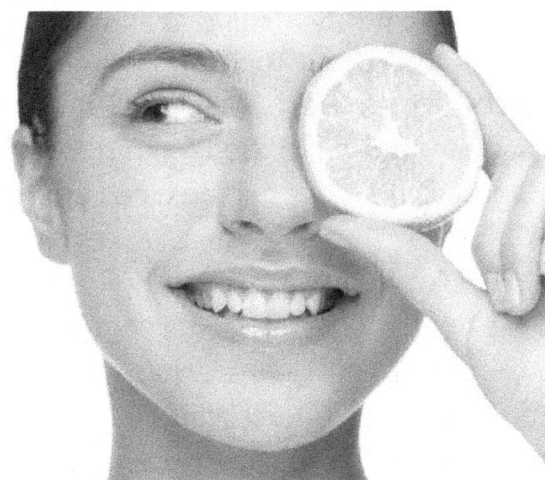

Juices

We will get to the good part in a bit – juices to use to keep you from fast aging and to maintain your youth. Juices should be the center of your health program. Many books and practitioners say that juices can harm you if used in excess. But juices and tonics are what you need to bring your health back to normal and to help you feel and be younger.

What is important in your health is what you eat. If you eat foods that harm you, you can look and feel 8 to 10 years older than you are. But if you eat and drink the right foods you can knock off 4 to 8 years off your appearance, in time.

In this e-book, you will find out how to use juices properly and for what purpose. In combination with vegetables and special anti-aging tonics and recipes, you will discover why juices of all types can reverse disease and help you maintain your young energy and appearance.

There are tremendous reasons to use a variety of juices and to find those tonics that provide unusual health benefits. Juice recipes are packed with minerals and special nutrients that can turn a sick body into one that is bursting with health. Choosing the right juice recipes are the key to do this.

Juice Tonics

Juice Tonics are special liquid mixtures that are designed to attack and reverse certain body ailments. In combination with juice recipes, they become a powerhouse to provide you with extraordinary anti-aging properties.

It is these juices and tonics that can provide you with the power to reverse your acid body into an alkaline body that can resist those diseases that are always nearby ready to take over your body. You can stop these diseases, but you have to know how to use the natural organic food that is available at many farmers market. If organic is not available, the next choices are to use non-organic but peel or wash them properly.

If you do not have fresh fruits or vegetables to use, then frozen is the next best choice. Frozen can be used in the blender to prepare juice or vegetable smoothies.

Using health tonics, smoothies, and special nutritional drinks are the best way to improve your health. No matter what illness you have, you need to incorporate these important drinks into your health routine.

The drinks you find here are some of the best mixtures you can find to help regain, maintain, and improve your health. These are not difficult drinks to make. Sometimes the ingredients may be a little bit difficult to find, but you can find them. It does require some persistence and motivation to be healthier and to leave discomfort, pain, and illness behind.

In these drinks, you will be using fruits, vegetables, vitamins, minerals, spices, herbs, and other special nutrients. All of these ingredients form one of the most powerful medicines you will ever find for stopping the degradation of your tissues, muscles, bones, and organs.

These juice recipes and tonics are considered life-saving and health promoting. Now, you can gain access to these drinks that you will be using forever and recommending to your friends and family. And, when you do, you will be doing them a great favor and giving the best health gift possible.

It is good to remember that drugs are good for helping you fight disease and injury. It is hard to do without some of these fine chemicals. But using them for a long time can be detrimental to your health. So as a compliment, you should always consider using juice recipes, tonics, and some smoothies with drugs so that you can slowly reduce their use and eventually eliminate them completely.

How You Maintain Youth

Most people think that to keep their youth and beauty you need to use topical creams or specially formulated creams that are advertised as anti-aging. This is the commercial side of anti-aging and does not provide you with a real long-term anti-aging program.

This book is not about special creams or face masks that you can apply on your skin to keep it from drying or wrinkling. It's about eliminating various body conditions or illnesses that can cause accelerated aging and that destroy your beauty and youthfulness prematurely. It is about stopping those body conditions that cause you inflammation and pain and prevent you from enjoying your life like you once did when you were young.

You cannot maintain outside beauty and youth if your insides do not have beauty and do not function properly. So the approach in the book is to help you get your insides working the way they should so that your outside reflects the beauty of your body insides. This is how you create and maintain beauty and youth and live a strong and useful life.

2: Why Juices Are Anti-Aging

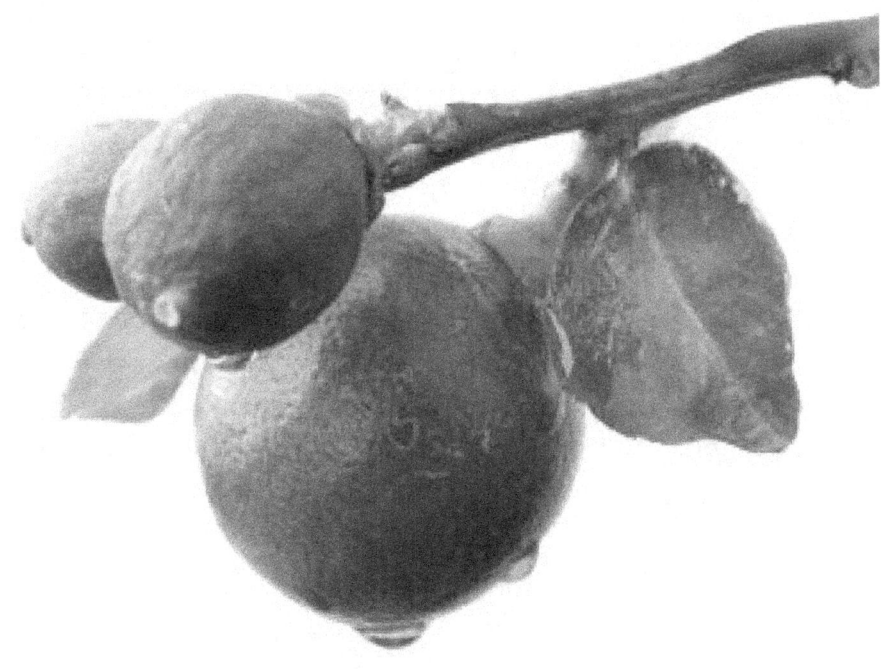

"Slow down the aging process by creating an alkaline body."

To slow down the aging process and maintain your beauty for more years than normal, you need to feed your body with the nutrients that it needs to function properly. When your body does not get what it needs, it starts the process of deterioration of the cells, tissue, bone, cartilage, muscles, and organs. It is this deterioration that makes you look older than you should.

So what is the first thing you need to do in this anti-aging program? You first need to know why you should start using the juices of fruits and vegetables.

From The Soil And Sun

Because fruits are naturally grown from the soil, they pull minerals of the ground and can have a great source of nutrients for you, if the soil is heavy with minerals. Because of these minerals and other nutrients, Fruits have amazing curative effects, when they are eaten raw. In some cases, it is better to cook them for their healing effects.

Because of plant photosynthesis, fruits and vegetables obtain the energizing frequencies that your body needs from the sun. This one of the reasons why raw has the power to maintain your youth. Raw contains the life you need in the variety of frequencies or colors that the sun provides.

As you eat these live produce, you absorb the live enzymes. Your cells obtain the energy of the nutrients which contain the energy expressed in the frequency of the sun. When you cook produce above 115 F, the life of the fruit or vegetable is destroyed and no longer has the full anti-aging value.

Alkaline Fruits

The best fruits to eat are those that allow your body to become more alkaline. Your body naturally seeks to be in an alkaline condition. In this condition, your body has less pain, inflammation, disease, and your appearance flourishes. Your body has more energy and it does not deteriorate as fast as when your body is filled with acid.

It's ok to eat fruits that make your body acid, but it best

to concentrate on the fruits that create alkalinity. This is because most people have an acid body and need to move it to an alkaline condition. Later, when you become more alkaline, you will be eating 80% alkaline fruits and 20% acid fruits.

Your body uses minerals to neutralize acids and to create simple or complex chemicals that your body needs. So, the body holds specific minerals in a certain way. It holds minerals in "storage" and releases them when they are needed for certain chemical reactions. The storage locations of minerals are in the blood, in organs, in cells, in tissue, in muscle and in the liquids inside and outside your cells.

Fruit Benefits

Fruits contain a variety of nutrients that are necessary for maintaining your life and beauty. Each nutrient has its function in the body. Many of the functions are known and many are not. Here is a list of some of the main known nutrients and what they do in your body.

- Minerals
- Antioxidants
- Phytonutrients
- Bioflavonoids
- Vitamins
- Enzymes

It is the following minerals and nutrients that contribute to giving you a youthful body.

Minerals

Your body contains around 4% minerals by weight.

Minerals have a lot of functions in the body. Your body's growth, development, and beauty depend on minerals. They act as partners with enzymes to work in your body to reduce inflammation. They provide structural support in bones and teeth, maintain water balance, and are involved in muscle contraction.

The condition of the interior of your body is reflected in your outer appearance. If your organs, tissue, bones, and cells do not receive the minerals they need, they are not able to regenerate themselves easily and start deteriorating. This poor health condition is reflected in your eye beauty, skin smoothness, hair fullness, joint flexibility, energy level, body pain, emotion healthiness, and your outlook on your life.

The minerals combine with other molecules to form complex ions such as hemoglobin. Maintaining a high level of oxygen in your body and cells is one of the secrets to maintain youth and fruits and vegetable help you get the maximum amount of oxygen your body needs.

Minerals are the secret key to helping you maintain alkaline-acid balance throughout your entire body. And, they assist in the transmission of information from the brain to within all body systems.

You didn't hear your mother saying, "take your minerals", normally you heard, "don't forget to take your vitamins." But minerals are one step above vitamins in that many vitamins cannot do their job in your body without minerals.

There are two types of minerals. First, there are regular minerals such as calcium, sodium, phosphorous, magnesium. These are the minerals you normally take daily.

Then there are trace minerals and these are like zinc, copper, arsenic, and iron. It's in the trace minerals that you can run the risk of mineral toxicity since you don't need much of these trace minerals. Of course, there are more minerals in each category. Here is a list of the major minerals you find in fruits.

Sodium, potassium, chloride, calcium, phosphorus, magnesium

Here is a list of the trace minerals:

Iron, selenium, zinc, copper, iodide, fluoride, chromium, manganese, molybdenum, boron, nickel, silicon, arsenic, vanadium

Minerals are found both in meat and in fruits and vegetables. Our concentration here is on minerals found in fruits and how they cure your body. Most all of these minerals are found in fruits, but there are some that are only found in meat and other foods.

There other minerals that are called heavy metals. These tend to displace other beneficial minerals and cause toxic effects. These metals are:
Lead, cadmium, mercury, arsenic, iron

Antioxidants

The body produces antioxidants to neutralize the free radicals that become excessive in our body. Free radicals have a damaging effect on the tissue, veins, and organs they encounter as they speed throughout your body. Left uncheck they cause numerous deadly diseases and destroy your youth.

The way the body takes care of this threat is to create antioxidants. However, the body's antioxidants are not always enough to capture and neutralize all these free radicals. This is because free radical can be created in numerous ways and can be found in food, air, water, and personal products.

Free radicals are also created by emotional states such as anger, fear, depression, and anxiety.

The result is that your body needs help to neutralize these free radicals, and this is where fruit and vegetable minerals come in. They are packed with antioxidants. Using them to neutralize free radicals has become a necessity.

There are many minerals and vitamins that are classified as antioxidants. These are vitamins A, C, E, and selenium. Other antioxidants are bioflavonoids, carotenoids, isoflavones, all minerals, allium vegetables like garlic and onions, bilberry, coenzyme Q10, cruciferous vegetables, ginkgo biloba, glutathione, lipoic acid, superoxide dismutase, and melatonin.

Phytonutrients

Phytochemicals or phytonutrients are mostly found

in the skin of fruits and are considered antioxidants. These nutrients give the fruit its color. Fruits also contain the fundamental antioxidants vitamin A, C, E, beta-carotene, zinc, and selenium. Try to buy organic fruits so you can eat the skins without worry. In some fruits, there are more nutrients on the skin than in the fruit.

Other antioxidants that you may have heard of are carotenoids, lutein, lycopene, sod, and glutathione, anthocyanins, and lipoic acid. The list is in the hundreds.

Phytonutrients found in fruits and other plants protect them from disease, insects, excess heat, UV rays, poisons, pollutants, injury, and drought.

Phytonutrients have been found to be beneficial to human life. They contain chemicals that are useful in treating and preventing diseases such as cancer, diabetes, cardiovascular disease, and hypertension.

The phytonutrients consist of many groups but the most important groups are the phytosterols and phytohormones. These sterols are precursors to your human sterols.

Bioflavonoids

Bioflavonoids are also antioxidants that are chemicals which come from water-soluble colors found in fruits, vegetables, grains, leaves, and barks. Because they are found in a variety of plant food they come in different chemical forms and concentrations.

Some of the bioflavonoids are more powerful in destroying free radicals then the standbys, vitamin C and E. Some well-known flavonoids are catechins, resveratrol, and proanthocyanidins.

Vitamins

Vitamins are needed in small amounts in your body to help it perform normal functions, to provide for growth and to assist in body maintenance. There are two types of vitamins, fat-soluble and water-soluble.

Most vitamins cannot be made in the body. Some can but in small amounts. For this reason, most vitamins that your body needs must come from the food you eat. Some fruits have vitamins. but they will not have all the vitamins your body needs.

Vitamins carry out various complex biochemical or physiological reactions in your body. When you lack the necessary vitamins your body needs, these chemical reactions do not occur often enough. The result is the creation of various illnesses and the loss of a youthful appearance. If the illnesses are not too far along, the illness can be reversed and your youthful energy retrieved.

As with all illness, if it is not too far along it can be reversed with the appropriate minerals, vitamins, or nutrients. In many cases, people wait too long before they address their illness. In some cases, people don't know they are ill or they just ignore that they don't feel good.

When it is reversible, then you need the foods that have the nutrients that will make you well and not the drugs that will keep or make you sick.

When you have an illness and wait too long to do something about it, you get tissue damage in your organs, veins, arteries, or body that is not reversible using natural methods. Your skin becomes spotty and wrinkled, your hair starts to thin, and your previous abundant energy is lost. Surgery or drugs can sometimes repair tissue damage, but you will not be the same as before when you were well.

3: The Anti-aging Power of Enzymes

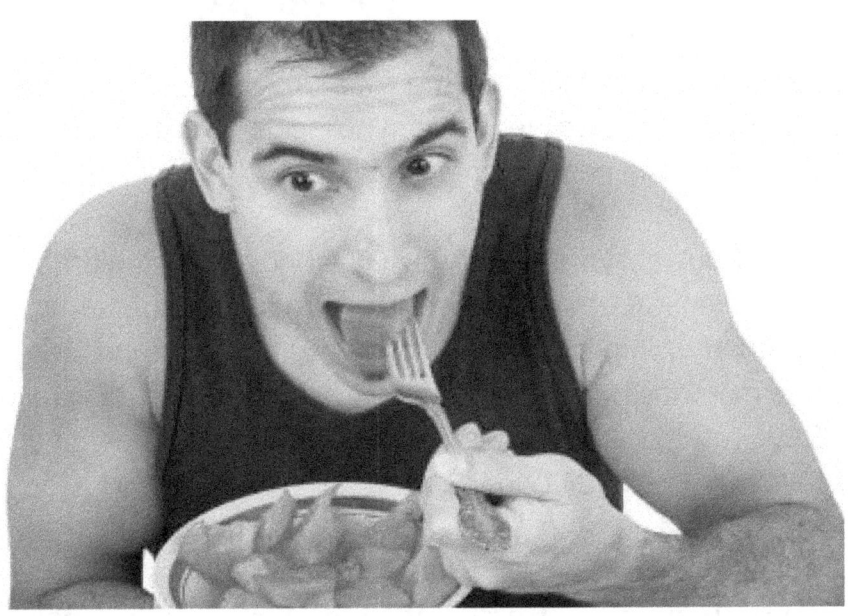

Enzymes

Enzymes need to be a priority in your anti-aging program. This is the best-kept secret to maintaining your youth and health. Using foods with plenty of enzymes or taking enzymes supplements is critical to slowing down your aging progress.

Enzymes have the ability to control and keep in check the oxidation process, which is the combination of oxygen and other substances. This combination causes the formation of free radicals and other substances that are detrimental to cells, tissue, and organs. This detrimental effect accelerates aging and you start to lose your beauty.

How Are Enzymes Made

Enzymes are composed of different amino acids connected together. The body can create many enzymes, but not all, because it uses amino acids in its links and not all amino acids are created in your body. There are some amino acids that only come from the food you eat. So you need to eat certain foods to get the amino acids your body needs to create all of the necessary enzymes.

Without enzyme activity in your body, you could not live. These chemical entities are required to help you breathe, give you energy, digest food, allow you to hear and see and perform thousands of other body activities. There are over 75,000 of these enzymes in your body and their chemical activity is constantly ongoing.

The body can only produce so many enzymes in your life. When you are sick, stressed, injured, depressed, or aged, you will produce less. This will cause you to become sick or sicker. Your appearance will change and you will look older than you are.

Getting Your Enzymes

You can also get enzymes from the raw food that you eat, which will supplement your body's enzymes. Enzymes are found in large quantities in fruits and vegetables. When food is processed and exposed to heat and encapsulated in a vacuum, the enzymes are destroyed.

Here is how you can maintain a high level of living

enzymes in your body and help yourself to a new level of youth.

Eat all your fruits and vegetables raw. If you have to cook fruits or vegetables, cook below 115F and just long enough to soften. If you don't have raw, then the next best is frozen produce. Freezing fruits temporarily inactivates enzymes. So you can use freeze produce in place of raw.

Use raw vegetables in a salad and use raw cold pressed wheat germ to increase your vitamin E intake.

Begin all of your meals with a salad. Doing this promotes the release of enzymes into your stomach to start the digestion process.

Try to use organic fruits and vegetable, when possible.

Start sprouting a variety of seeds because they contain powerful enzymes and are abundant in minerals.

You can use raw milk, cream, or buttermilk. These are usually not available in the US, but some stores may have them. They are packed with enzymes

Create seeds that you can sprout through a coffee mill to create a powder. Mix the powder with a liquid like milk, water, or juice to create a drink. Use only those seeds that are alive and can be sprouted. This drink will be packed with enzymes.

If you need to cook produce, use a temperature below 115 F.

All fruits have enzymes that help you digest them. This is why it is best to eat them raw and benefit from the natural enzymes. Eating fruits raw instead of cooked, in cans, in bottles, or in any other processed package saves your own body's enzymes.

When you are sick, drinking fresh juices helps your immune system in that it does not have to use up its own enzymes, which are used up in fighting your disease.

Your body has only a certain number of enzymes that it can produce in your lifetime. That is why after a certain age it is best to start taking digestive enzymes with each meal. But it is also wise to take digestive enzymes at any age. These supplements provide a safety net to preserve your vitality and young appearance.

Lack of digestive enzymes causes poor nutrition. Most elderly have poor nutrition and are very weak because they don't use digestive enzymes. In addition as you age, your stomach Hydrochloric acid, HCl, decreases and at some point in time you would need to supplement with digestive enzymes with HCl acid. You need good HCL in your stomach to transform some of the minerals and vitamins from the food you eat.

4: How Fruit Minerals Burn Acid

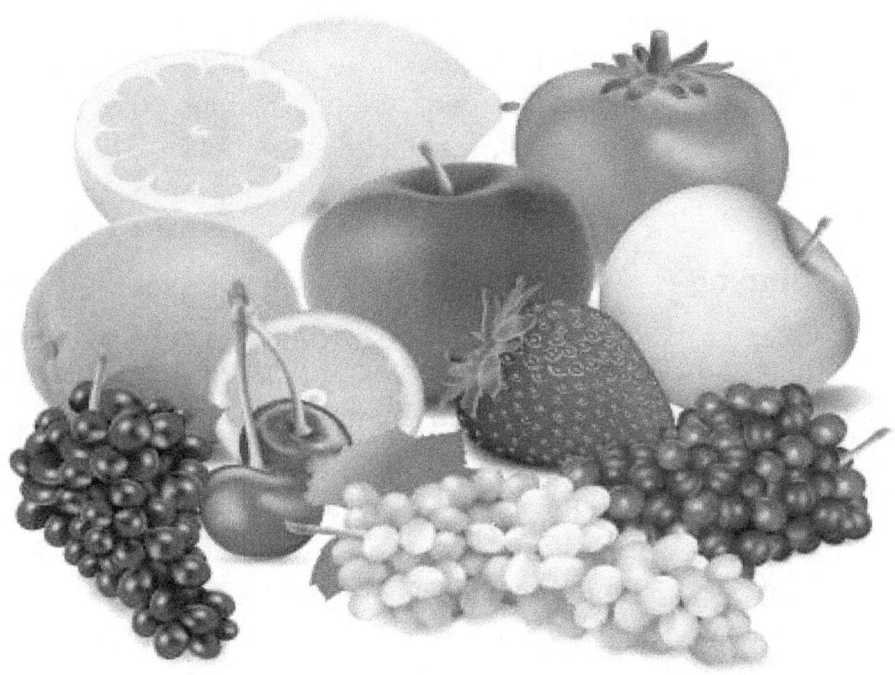

Minerals

Moving your body more toward alkalinity is what will give you the best curative effects of fruits. An alkaline body prevents your body from becoming ill and forming deadly diseases, like all kinds of joint problems, organ degradation, body pain, or even cancer. If you are already sick, then all of the chemicals inside fruits will help to revive you to better health. This is provided that your tissue damage has not gone beyond repair.

The minerals of most importance in changing and maintaining your body in an alkaline condition are sodium, potassium, chloride, calcium, phosphorus, magnesium, and sulfur.

Now how your body can become alkaline might become a little confusing at first because of the terms used, but let's break this down into small parts. First, we are going to be defining some terms so we can then start talking the same language.

Acid Binding

There are certain minerals that are called acid binding. And these are minerals we said are the most important ones in fruits, Sodium, potassium, chloride, calcium, phosphorus, magnesium, because they are acid binding.

What acid binding means is when you eat fruits with these minerals, they will seek out acids in your body and combine with them to neutralize them by creating a new chemical called alkaline forming ash.

Alkaline Ash

Now this alkaline forming ash has tied up acid and is now carried to the kidney where it is expelled as urine.

Different reactions can occur when an acid-binding mineral, like say sodium, encounters an acid. Of course, acids in the body are toxic, so the body has the priority of getting rid of them fast since they can damage tissue and cause pain and disease.

Here is another pathway of the acid-binding mineral process, when it combines with an acid.

The Acid Binding Mineral Process

When you eat acid binding food, the blood carries it to the cells where it is oxidized, digested, or metabolized. The result of this digestion is a carbonic acid salt of alkaline minerals, which reacts with body acids and bind with them. In this process, weak carbonic acid is created. Now, this weak carbonic acid is taken by the blood into the lungs where it is released as carbon dioxide and water.

If not all the acid toxins are captured by acid binding matter, the remaining acids can be neutralized by body stores of alkaline minerals. If you don't have a good store of alkaline minerals, then these acids will remain in your body creating disease. But if you do have a good store of alkaline minerals, then these minerals will find these acids, capture them and bind with them. Then these acids are routed out through your urine and out of your body.

So you can see the importance of getting a lot of alkaline minerals into your body. Without them, acids which do not get bonded to alkaline minerals would move back into body tissue and continue their body damage.

Alkaline Binding

Now, there are also minerals that become alkaline binding and these minerals are sulfur, chlorine, iodine, phosphorous, bromine, fluorine, copper, and silicon.

It is these minerals that when digested by a cell will produce a salt that will bind with alkaline minerals. These minerals will be excreted through your urine. When alkaline minerals are bonded to an acid salt, the alkaline mineral is removed from your body and your body becomes more acidic, the condition you are trying to avoid.

Although you need to eat both foods that are acid binding or alkaline binding, you want to eat more of the acid-binding foods.

Keeping Healthy

One of the most important parts of health is keeping the lymph liquid around your cells clean and free of toxins. To do this you need to provide alkaline minerals to occupy the lymph liquid and you need to remove the acids that accumulate in that liquid and in all parts of your body tissue. You can do this by detoxifying your body and providing alkaline minerals for lymph liquid.

Body Detoxification

The highest priority of the body is to detoxify itself. One of the best way to help your body detoxify is to provide minerals that bind with acids that are in the cells, tissues, organs, and muscles. What these alkaline acid binding minerals do is to pull out the toxins that are dispersed throughout your body. These acid binding salts have the ability to suck those acids out and bind with them. But, because not all body chemical reactions follow the same directions there are times that the alkaline acid binding does not take place.

With the help of the liver which detoxifies the blood, the kidney that removes impurities from the blood and the lungs which removes the CO 2, which results from alkaline acid binding, your body is constantly detoxifying itself. But when it is overloaded with acid toxins from your lifestyle, a complete detox of your body become impossible.

Where do Acid Toxins Come From

So why is the body overloaded with toxins? Why can't the liver take care of these toxins? The liver has the function to remove acid wastes from natural food that is created by food digestion and cell metabolism. When it encounters acid wastes such as food enhancers, dyes, preservatives, pesticides, and the variety of additives, the liver does not know how to break them down and to make them harmless.

Your body does not give up so easily when it knows that the liver was not able to disintegrate food additives. What it does is it instructs calcium to bind with these toxic acids and to take them far away from the bloodstream. The result is that calcium binding with acid forms a deposit and this deposit can be placed in your teeth, your joints, and as bone spurs, which grow in your feet or shoulders, vertebra, or muscle tissue. These calcium deposits are very painful, and if you have ever experienced them, you know how much.

Now, we have talked about acid toxins in the body that are brought in through food and the environment. But there is another factor that creates acid in the body and that is emotions that are activated through life stresses, like work pressures, divorce, friendship problems, marital issues, and other similar problems. These emotional problems create acidic molecules that then embed themselves into your tissues just like food acids.

Body Organs

All body organs function to rid the body of acid waste or toxins. Lack of alkaline binding food causes deterioration of the function of these organs. Each organ has a specific function in the elimination and neutralization of acid wastes and it does this in conjunction with alkaline acid binding minerals.

5: Fruits to Eat And Drink To Preserve Youth

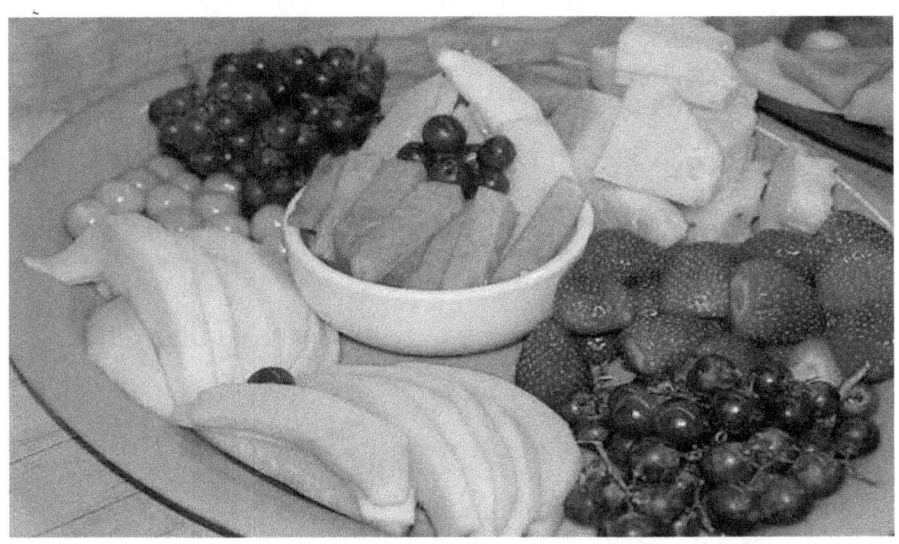

Below are the fruits to eat and drink that you need to concentrate on to make your body alkaline. You can prepare fresh juices from these fruits and receive the power of minerals that combine with your body acid to give and protect your youth and beauty. This is the most powerful anti-aging therapy you can give yourself.

When you eat fruits, your cells digest or metabolize the fruit nutrients and leave behind free radicals. Antioxidants neutralize these free radicals. Free radicals attack internal cell material, cell membrane, and tissue, creating inflammation and all kinds of diseases. Antioxidants are the main natural remedy for preventing arteriosclerosis, coronary heart disease, senility, aging, cancer, cataracts, and many other inflammatory diseases.

Fruits

1. **Fruits at 100% Acid Binding – Best fruits To Eat**
   Lemons, melons – any type, watermelon

2. **Fruits at 93% Acid Binding – Great fruits To Eat**
   Cantaloupes, dried dates, dried figs, limes, mango, papaya

3. **Fruits at 87% Acid Binding – Still Great Fruits To Eat**
   Kiwis, passion fruit, pineapples, raisins, umeboshi plums

4. **Fruits at 80% Acid Binding – Eat These Fruits**
   Apricots, avocados, bananas, fresh dates, fresh figs, currants, gooseberries grapes, grapefruits guavas, kumquats, nectarines, pears, persimmons, quince, berries, cactus

5. **Fruits at 73% Acid Binding – Still Fruits To Eat**
   Apples, oranges, peaches, pomegranate, raspberries, sour grapes, strawberries, carob

6. **Fruits at 67% Acid Binding – Still Neutralizes Acids**
   Cherries, fresh coconut

7. **Herbal Teas From Leaves at 73% to 86% acid binding**

Alfalfa, mint, sage, spearmint, raspberry strawberry comfrey

8. **All Herbs and Spices at 67% to 73% Acid Binding**

9. **Fruits At 40% to 47% - Eat less of these fruits**

    Blueberries, cranberries, plums, prunes

All fruit juices from a juicer 100% acid binding

6: Fruit Juices That Create Youth & Health

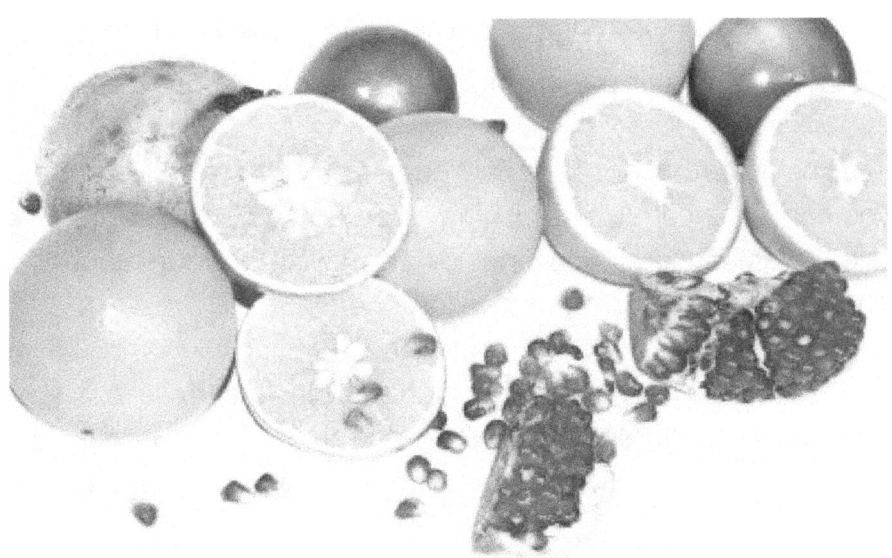

Eating fruits whole, blended, or as juices is what creates heath. In this chapter may juices recipes are given, but you should also eat these fruits whole or blended to get the fiber they contain.

Teeth Lemon Juice Recipe

For bleeding gums, rub the rind part of lemon along your bleeding gums each day. Use this as long as you have bleeding.

Teeth Whitening

For a teeth whitening, use a combination of fresh lemon,

lime, and grapefruit juice and brush your teeth and leave it on without rinsing your mouth. Do this three times a week.

Toothache

For a toothache, use a cotton soak in lemon juice and put it on top or side of the aching tooth for a few minutes.

For a toothache, bleeding gums, or any teeth discomfort, you can do coconut oil swishing. You do this by each morning take a tablespoon of coconut oil and swish in your mouth for 10 to 15 minutes. Do not swallow the oil.

After the time is up, spit out the oil, and rinse out your mouth with a little bit of salt and water. Then brush your teeth normally. Do this for 1 to 2 weeks and see how it improves your mouth health.

The health of your mouth is central to your overall health since it has been found that mouth bacteria can enter your bloodstream and affect your various body organs.

Sore throat

For a sore throat, you can gargle with lemon juice a few times a day. This gargle can also be done with apples cider vinegar. I usually dilute the lemon or apple cider vinegar slightly. Use around 1 oz. of apple cider or lemon juice to 6 oz. of distilled water. Or you can try a stronger version of 50:50 apple cider vinegar.

In the **Fruit Chart** given above, you will see that the fruit that gives you the best acid binding in your cells is Lemon. It is high in potassium and calcium and is low in the minerals that produce acid – phosphorus, chlorine, and sulfur. Also notice it only takes 1 1/2 hours to digest, which helps you in the morning to detoxify your liver, blood, and cells.

Insomnia

Lemons can be used for insomnia. Prepare a drink using lemon and orange juice, honey and hot water. Drink this just before going to bed.

Another drink that can help you sleep is preparing a banana and milk in a blender. You can drink this about ½ hour before going to bed.

Getting the right amount of sleep, 7 to 8 hour, will keep you looking young and will extend your lifespan.

Hemorrhoid Fig Juice Recipe

Boil fig leaves in 8 oz. of distilled water. Put under low heat and continue to boil until you have 4 oz. or half the liquid you started with.

Apply the liquid to the anus, using a cotton ball.

Grapes – Grapes are filled with phytochemicals. They contain resveratrol, ellagic acid, quercetin, and some phytosterols. Because of these phytochemicals, grapes are at the top of the list for fighting free radical. This also puts grapes at the top of the list for producing long life and beauty.

Doctors have found that drinking 10 ounces of purple grape juice a day will make blood platelets less sticky. This means blood clots, which can lead to heart attacks, are less likely to occur.

Grape juice is more effective than aspirin in reducing the formation of blood clots.

For the skin, use green Thompson seedless. Just cut the grape slightly and rub the juice into the area where you want to reduce wrinkles. You can also blend these grapes and put this mash of grapes on your face and leave them on for 15 to 22 minutes.

Guavas – This fruit is high in lycopene, an antioxidant, and is a good source of Vitamin C. This fruit is great for lowering high blood pressure and cholesterol levels.

Ripe guavas can be used as a tonic for making weak hearts stronger. In addition, eating guavas helps to overcome lung and throat congestion.

Guava Juice For Diabetes

Its juice has been used to control diabetes. Drink the juice right before a meal to control the sugar spikes that might come from that meal.

Mangoes - Mango, and papaya are also high on the alkaline ash list so include that as snacks between meals and drink their juices.

Retinopathy Mango Juice Tonic

For eye blood vessels that are weak due to diabetic retinopathy make a tea from mango leaves.

Steep mango leaves for an hour

Filter this liquid

Combined with a couple tablespoons of mango or pineapple

Drink this combination twice a day.

Now drink this combination.

Papayas – This fruit contains a protein digestive enzyme called papain. Papain is available in tablets in many health food stores. It has been found that papain has the ability to neutralize snake poisons resulting from snake bites.

Poison Snake Papaya Juice Recipe

By taking 5 tablets with 1 teaspoonful of Adolph's meat tenderizer dissolved in a cup of warm water within 30 minutes of a bite, a person has the chance of surviving a venous bite are good.

Peaches – Red peaches are a great source of beta-carotene coupled with vitamin C and fiber. Cooking peaches makes them lose a lot of their fiber.

If you want a facial mask made of peaches for skin rejuvenation, here's what to do. In a blender mix peach, papaya, banana, and avocado, then place this mixture on your face for 30 minutes. Afterward, put some natural oil on your face like virgin coconut oil, or sunflower oil and expect better skin texture than before.

7: The Power of Vegetable To Keep You, Young

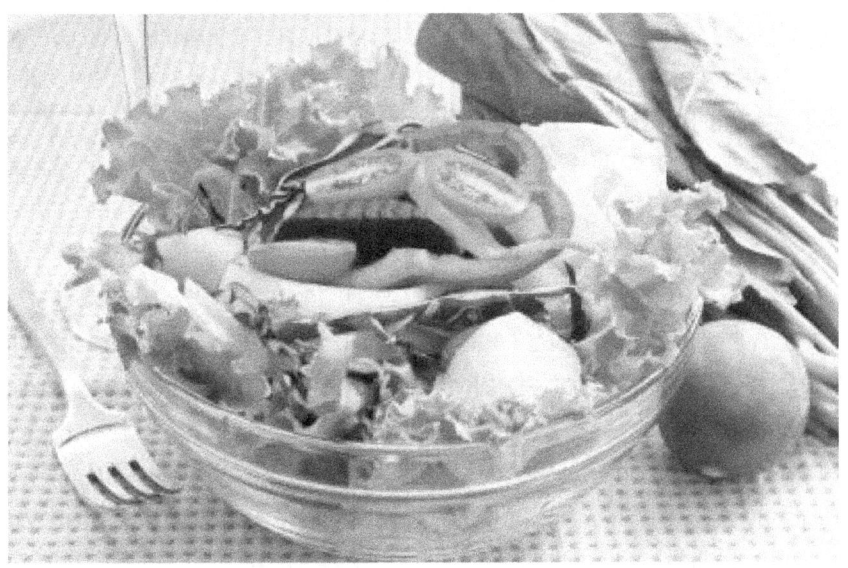

Vegetable Power

Vegetables have the power to bring your body back into the normal range of health. This is because many of the acid you produce during the day, vegetables can neutralize them. If you do not neutralize these acids, they build up in your body and attract and create disease. Your body will age faster when it is filled with acid.

The number of diseases that result from an acid buildup in your body encompasses practically all diseases.

Body Acids Reabsorbed

If body acids, which are created during cell digestion, are not neutralized or eliminated, they will be reabsorbed and distributed throughout your body. These acids go from the colon into the bloodstream and then into the liver. Then, from there they get back into your lymph liquid and deposit themselves into your body tissues.

Mineral Binding

The only way to reduce the detrimental effects of these acids on your body is to mix them with an alkaline liquid. This is where fruits and vegetables come in. They have the power to provide what is known as "mineral binding", which helps to neutralize the effect of excess body acids or excess alkaline compounds. But in this e-book, we are mainly concerned with the toxic acids that you have in your body.

In addition to reducing or eliminating an acidic body condition, vegetables contain 100's of chemicals known and unknown. The chemicals are minerals, vitamins, phytonutrients, antioxidants, bioflavonoids, and other natural nutrients.

It's these different chemicals that help you to cure certain body ills. The thing to remember, when using vegetables to cure, is you have to use more of them compared to when you are just eating them for breakfast, lunch or snacks. When you have an acid body, you are short on minerals that bind to the body's acid waste.

Natural Salicylates

Studies have shown that people who eat plenty of vegetables and fruits have less cancer and heart disease. It has been found that people who eat these foods have high levels of salicylates in their blood, even though they do not use aspirin. These natural salicylate chemical have an anti-inflammatory effect, which provides a reduction in inflammatory diseases.

Inflammation is one of the conditions that are associated with accelerated aging. Inflammation causes a slow deterioration of the whole body. You can a low-level inflammation which works slowly and unknowingly in your body creating a disease that shows up when you are older.

Disease Fighting

We all know that vegetables have a lot of vitamins, minerals, and special nutrients. This produce is one of the main sources of fiber that is critical for your health. But vegetables have another set of nutrients that we should take advantage of and these are called Phytochemicals.

Phytochemicals are found in plants are responsible for the plants color, smell, and other qualities of the plant. It is these chemicals that most likely are able to affect, eliminate or cure various diseases.

Many drugs have been created by extracting certain chemicals from plants and producing pills in mass.

Unfortunately, drugs that are created are unbalanced and unlike the vegetables, they came from. The results are side effects that you need to endure as you use these pills.

Vegetables contain all the vitamins, minerals and nutrient in the proper balance or ratios. That is why you seldom get sick when you eat vegetables.

Knowing which vegetable to use for sickness and disease is important. When you use vegetables for illness, you need to use much more than what you eat at mealtime. In this e-book, you will discover some of the vegetable cures that you should know about and be using to help yourself or your family.

Here are the vegetables you should be eating and drinking

Vegetables

Here is the list of vegetables to eat in order of priority. All of these vegetables will neutralize acid, since they contain minerals that are acid binding.

10. Vegetables at 93% Acid Binding – best vegetables to eat

    Kelp, Seaweed, Watercress, Asparagus

11. Vegetables at 80% Acid Binding – Still the best to eat

    Lettuce Leaf, Oyster plant, Pumpkin, Spinach, Squash, Peas, Carrots, Celery, Chard, Swiss, Dandelion greens

12. Vegetables at 73% Acid Binding – Great vegetables to eat

    Bamboo shoots, Beets, Broccoli, Cabbage, Cauliflower, Collards, Corn, sweet, Ginger (fresh), Mushrooms, Mustard greens, Onions, Pepper, Potatoes, Green, Lima, String, Potatoes

13. Vegetables at 67% Acid Binding – eat plenty of these

    Brussels sprouts, Cucumbers, Eggplant, Okra, Onions, Radishes, Tomatoes

14. Vegetable juices at 80% to 93% Acid Binding

    Parsley, wheatgrass, carrot, celery, etc.

15. Soy Bean Products at 60% Acid Binding – Limit your use of tofu since it is a genetically modified organism, GMO

    Dried beans, Soy cheese, Soy milk, Tempeh, Tofu

More Acid Binding Food

Here are some other misc. foods to eat that are acid binding. Using acid binding foods of all kinds should be in your arsenal against the ravishes of body acids and free radicals.

16. Starches at 80% Acid Binding

    Arrowroot flour

17. Sugar at 73% acid Binding

    Honey

18. Nuts and Seeds at 60 % to 67% Acid Binding

Almonds, sesame seeds, Granola, Essene Bread, Chestnuts

19. Misc. foods at 60% Acid Binding

Horseradish, Amaranth, Millet, Quinoa, Dried beans, Soy cheese, Soy milk,

The following foods are Alkaline binding, which means that they create acids that will bind with alkaline salts and remove them from your body. These foods, when eaten in excess, will create an acid body. You should only eat around 20% of these foods in your diet and the other 80% should come from fruits and vegetables or foods that are acid binding. When you eat with this 20/80 formula, you will have an alkaline body.

NOTE: The lower the alkaline binding percentage, the more that food is acid producing.

20. All oils are basically at 50% and are considered neutral.

This includes almond, avocado, canola, coconut, corn castor, olive, soy, sunflower oil, and etc.

21. Beans, starches, and nuts and seeds at 40% to 46% Alkaline Binding

Aduki, Black, Broadbean, Garbanzo, Mung, Pinto, Barley, Corn Meal, Lentils, Brans, Cashews, Coconut (dried), Pecans, Brans, Millet, Filberts, Walnuts, Pumpkin, Sunflower

22. **Starches at 26 to 33 % Alkaline Binding**

Brown Rice, Buckwheat, Oats, Spelt, Wheat Whole, Peanuts, corn, rye

23. **Rice at 20% Alkaline Binding**

White rice

24. **Sugar at 13% Alkaline Binding**

White beet or cane sugar

Meat and Fish

25. **Meat at 26% alkaline binding**

Fish With fins and scales, Shellfish - shrimp, scallops, crab lobster, oyster

26. **Meat at 20% Alkaline Binding**

Chicken, turkey, rabbit

27. **Meat at 13% Alkaline Binding**

Beef, goat, pork, lamb

28. **All oils are basically at 50% and are considered neutral.**

This includes almond, avocado, canola, coconut, corn castor, olive, soy, sunflower oil, and etc.

29. **Misc. Products at 13% to 26% Alkaline Binding**

Liquor, wine, beer, coffee, black tea, caffeine drinks

8: What You Should Know About Vegetable Juices

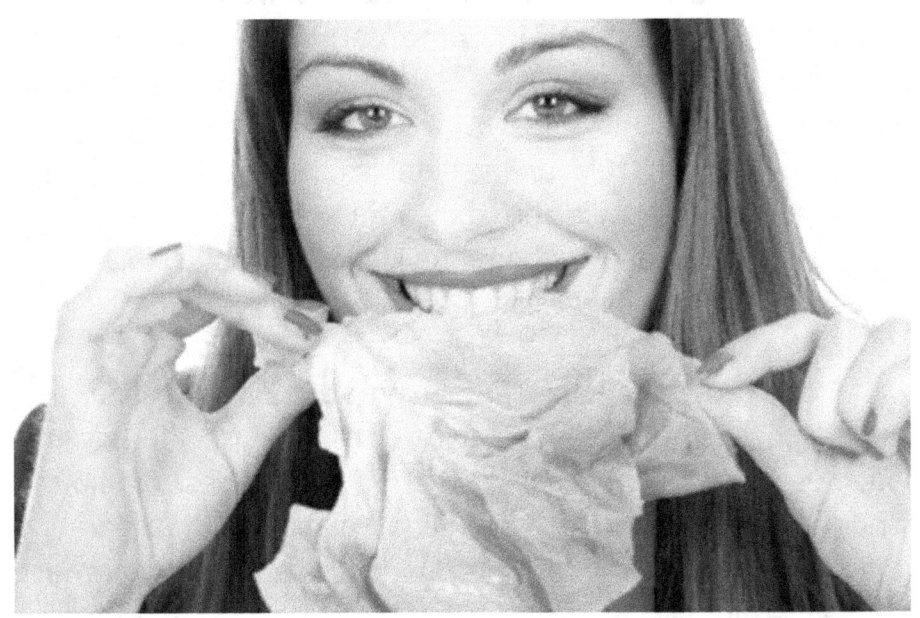

"Creating the best health requires is a lot of work. It requires persistent and dedication."

In this chapter, you will discover the curative power of vegetable juices. Vegetables contain all the nutrients that are necessary to feed every cell, tissue, organ, and bone in your body. They contain all of the vitamins, minerals, and nutrients necessary to repair, rebuild and create new cell structures. With the variety of nutrients that they have, they can replenish and rebuild the various organs in your body. They contain the nutrients that will prevent, stop, and cure all diseases.

The water in vegetables is both cleansing and curative. The minerals they contain will help to alkalinize your body.

"The continuous and persistent practice of getting the liquid life of fruits and vegetables into the system is one of the secrets of keeping young ..." Dr. Paul Bragg

Because fresh fruits and vegetables contain around 70% water, just as our bodies do, they are the perfect food to eat and drink. The water in them provides your body with cleansing and nutritional power.

Fresh vegetable juices have high nutritional, healing, and curing powers. Using vegetable juices as juice therapy has been used throughout the world and for centuries to help the body recover from nearly everybody aliment. By separating the juice from its fiber, its minerals and nutrients are suspended in the distilled water of the juice. This allows for your body to digest and absorb vegetable juice within minutes as compared with hours when eating the entire vegetable.

The actual amount of vitamins, minerals, and nutrients in vegetables that are grown in different states and countries will vary depending on the soil condition. To get the best nutrition, always chose the vegetables grown in your area and in season.

The value of fresh vegetable juices lies in the enzymes that they have. Enzymes are the source of life for your body since they provide the vibration or energy for other body chemical reactions to occur. Enzymes are used in most body chemical reactions and in the digestion of food. They are catalysts and they promote chemical action or change without changing their own status or state. If fruits, vegetables, seeds, or nuts are subject to temperatures from 115 F to 125 F, their enzymes start to slow down. At the temperature of 130 F, the enzymes are destroyed and no longer active.

Drinking fresh juices, especially when you are sick, is one way to recover faster from illness. Vegetable juices digest quicker than then the actual raw vegetable. The digestion of vegetables takes time and energy. The energy to digest the vegetable comes from the vegetable itself. When you are sick, you need to preserve your energy or allow your immune system to use the energy you have to fight off disease. You need to drink more juices when you are sick than when you are not.

When you are **not** sick, you can use juices to maintain your health. You use juices not as a substitute for your regular meals, but in conjunction with them. Juices provide quick energy with the natural sugar they contain, which is used right away by your body. But when you feel light-headed or dizzy, you can drink 3 oz. of grape, prune, apple or pineapple juice to eliminate the dizziness. These juices help to bring oxygen to your brain which stops the dizziness.

They provide a good supply of enzymes that are used to process the juice and for other body chemical reactions. When you provide your body with external enzymes - as with fresh juices or by supplementation - you preserve your body's enzymes for other necessary and more important chemical reactions in your organs and blood. When you eat dead food, not raw fruits, vegetables, and their juices, your body has to create and provide the enzymes necessary to digest this dead food. Dead food is any food that does not have enzymes and this includes fruits and vegetables that are cooked above 115 F to 130 F.

Using vegetable juice in correcting, healing or curing illness can have some side effects when they are used with people that are **using drugs.** Short-term side effects may be expected, but extend ones indicate that the juice you are using maybe the wrong type or amount. It is always best to work with a nutritionist or doctor when using juices as therapy with people using drugs, to ensure side effects can be counterbalanced with adjustments in the juices.

When you are not using drugs, then juices are safe and have few side effects other than those effects that result from your body excreting toxins. As toxins are released from various cells, tissue or organs a feeling of uneasiness or nausea can occur. But this will pass as the toxins being removed decrease. The duration of this sick feeling will depend on your level of toxicity. If the feeling of nausea is excessive, back off on the number of juices your use and increase them little by little.

Try to get fresh and organic vegetables, at farmers markets, when juicing. Many of the vegetables you find at the grocery store, especially if it is off-season for these vegetables, have been cold stored and sprayed with pesticides and have lost their nutritional value.

Using vegetable juice to diminish, eliminate or cure

disease requires that correct juice application. Reduce the use of meat, starchy, fried, greasy, and spicy foods when you are sick. This makes the vegetable and fruit juices more powerful in curing disease and creating the youth that you want.

The main idea in using vegetable juices is using light, juicy, juices, which provide for physical needs, correct metabolism, and improve general well-being. Juices should not be boring and should satisfy taste and hunger.

Using Vegetable Juices

Consider vegetable drinks like a meal. They should not be drunk with a meal or with any other food. You can add brewer's yeast, vitamin C powder, or acidophilus powder to them. You can take digestive enzymes with those juices that are not fresh and that come in a can, bottle, or are frozen.

Avoid those vegetable juices that are high in salt content. If you are drinking tomato juice, drink only that juice that is 100% tomato.

You can mix certain juices together to get a better taste. You can use the pulp from juicing vegetables to thicken soups or for a compost pile.

If you don't like to eat vegetables or if you are sick and need to recover, then juicing is the ideal way to get nutrients into your body. Juicing vegetables is another way to get the benefits of vegetables without eating them. Juicing them does not get you the entire benefit of the whole vegetable.

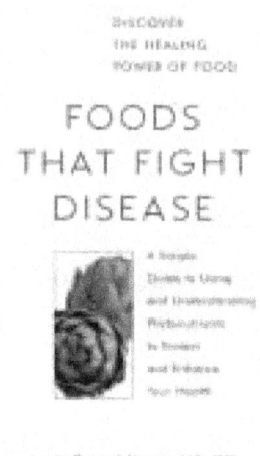

In Her book, Mozian, Deutsch, Laurie, M.S., R.D., Foods That Fight Disease, Penguin Putnam Inc., 2000, she says, "Juicing fresh fruits and vegetables gives you the ability to boost your intake of certain phytochemicals in a package most closely resembling what nature provides. A study examined the fate of three phytochemicals – beta-carotene, lycopene, and sulforaphane – during the process of juicing determined that juicing delivers about 1/2 of the important phytochemicals present in the original food. The remainder is discarded with the pulp. Some, however, would argue that getting 50% of a nutrient is better than getting none of it."

How Much Juice You Should Drink

A general guideline for drinking juice is as follows:

Use eight oz. if you are over 140 lbs.

Use 6 oz. if you weight 110 to 140 lbs.

Use 4 oz. if you are under 110 lbs.

If you are sick then you want to take at least 3 times this amount. And you spread this over the day. To maintain your youth you should be using at least 2x this amount and at the same time be eating the fruits that come in the top of the acid-binding list in a later chapter.

If you have diabetes, then you want to limit the amount of juices you drink, since they are normally high in sugar. But for many people, drinking juices is ok, since it may be the only way they will eat vegetables.

Drinking an excess of fresh vegetable and even fruit juices are not recommended. When you need to get nutrients fast into your body, when you are sick, then plenty of juice makes sense. If you are doing a body cleanse with juices, then it makes sense. But to drink half a gallon or more of juices of any kind when you are healthy, then this does not make sense.

Juicing gives you half of the vegetable. It is not a natural food. Drinking an excess of juices puts a strain on the liver and pancreas, which quickly has to restore your blood sugar levels. The amount of sugar your body can naturally process is the amount of sugar you find in whole vegetables and fruits. Without fiber, the juices are absorbed quickly into your body causing a spike in your blood sugar level. With fiber from the produce, you will absorb the sugar from the produce much slower.

9: The Cures From Vegetable Juice

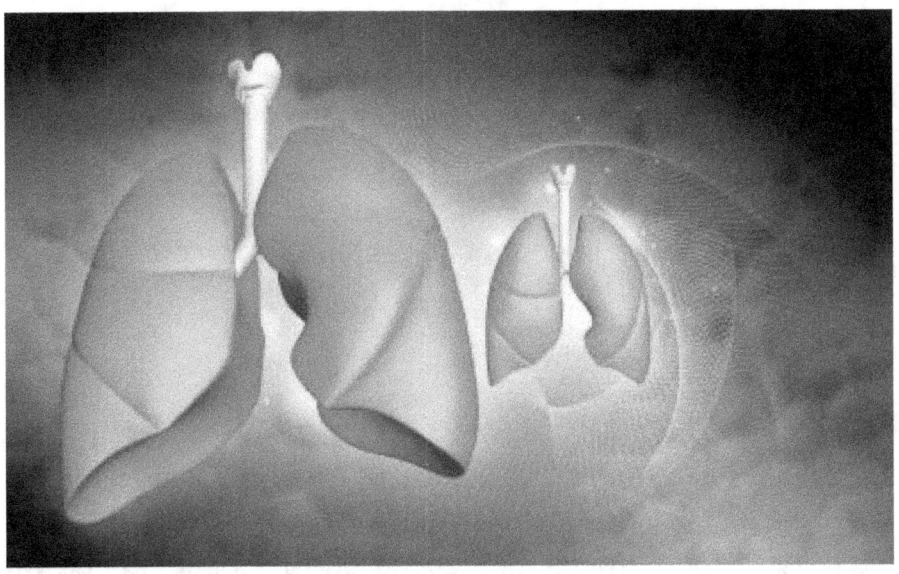

Juices are good to complement your daily nutritional program. Using many glasses of various juices daily should be reserved for therapeutical reasons.

In this chapter, you will find how various juices either by themselves or in combination with other juices give you curative powers. Whenever you are sick or are sick for a long time your youth is slipping away from you. To maintain your youth and beauty, you need to strive for good health in all parts of your body. When you have arthritis, you will age faster. When you have hair loss, you will lose some of your beauty. So to keep your beauty, the secrets are to maintain the best health possible. Any sick organ or part of your body will bring your beauty and youth down, sometimes fast and sometimes slowly.

Even though you feel you are not sick or don't have any body issues or conditions, then you still need to follow a healthy living. Drinking those acid binding juices fills your body stores with minerals that are used up daily and this is what keeps the beauty and youth that give you a fun filled life.

Here are some important juices and their corresponding healing powers:

Alfalfa Juice

Alfalfa has an array of great vitamins – A, C, K, and P – and over 21 trace and natural minerals. Of course, the actual intensity of the nutrient will depend on the soil it was grown in. This is one of the best juices to drink to alkalize your body. One of the best ways to drink this juice is to buy alfalfa powder.

Allergies Alfalfa Juice Recipe

Take powdered alfalfa and combine it with oranges, lemon, grapefruits, or pineapple juice. Choose the juices that fit your taste.

1 tablespoon of alfalfa power

8 oz. of carrot or tomato juice

Squeeze in 1/2 lemon juice

Place in a blender and blend for a minute or so

It best to use alfalfa power with a vegetable juice, but you can also use a citrus juice or pineapple. Experiment with different juices and find the one you like. When you drink this juice, it suggested that you take one capsule of enzymes.

Alfalfa has chemicals called saponins, which are detergent-like compounds. It is these compounds that can scrub the internal surfaces of your arteries to remove plaque and to prevent its build up. Alfalfa helps you reduce the devastating effects of arteriosclerosis.

In cases where you have symptoms of an acid body, alfalfa is what you need. Gout is a result of acid compounds created by eating an excess of meat and not eating enough vegetables. Alfalfa with its high levels of alkaline minerals will eliminate gout.

Ulcer Aloe Vera Juice Recipe

Aloe vera juice is a high powered juice. This juice is used for soothing the bowel area when it is irritated.
If you have hemorrhoids it can provide you some relief.
Here's how to use it.

There are some aloe vera juice drinks that you can buy at a health food store. Try them out and see what your results are. If you have the aloe jell then,

Mix 1-2 tablespoons with 7up or some other carbonated drink. Try different aloe portions until you find one that is palatable.

Also, mix Aloe with different juices until you find one that tastes good to you.

Aloe vera juice is also good if you have an ulcer or some internal lining scratch or tear. Aloe promotes the repair and regrowth of cells.

Weight Loss Artichoke, Jerusalem Juice Recipe

This juice is well known for controlling weight. It does this when this juice is used in a certain way. Artichokes have a high amount of inulin. This is not like insulin but is a carbohydrate that moves quickly into your bloodstream to provide energy for the liver, spleen, and pancreas to help stabilize and normalize your sugar levels. This is a good juice for chronic fatigue syndrome, hypoglycemia, and diabetes.
Juice artichoke in your juicer
Mix this juice with carrot juice 1:1.

Add one tablespoon of alfalfa powder

Mix this juice with equal parts of carrot, alfalfa or beet juice.

For a weight loss program, drink this juice through a straw and swish it around in your mouth before swallowing. This helps to reduce your cravings for sweets or junk food.

Kidney Asparagus Juice

Asparagus has an alkaloid call Asparagine in high amounts. Asparagine is a non-essential amino acid. Alkaloids are compounds mostly found in plants and some are good and some are poison. In this case, Asparagine is beneficial for the body. It is an alkaline food and it has been found that the nervous system needs it for proper functioning.

If you do not get it in food, your body will create it. The only way to get this alkaloid into your body is by drinking asparagus juice. When you cook asparagus, this nutrient is lost.

Pure asparagus juice is quite strong and you should mix it with carrot juice. Or Combine it with beet, carrot and cucumber juice.

This juice is used as a diuretic and is used for kidney dysfunctions. Its juice is capable of breaking up kidney oxalic stones. It has a history of curing patients with acute nephritis or Bright's disease, a severe kidney disease.

This juice is good for cancer, eye disorders, gout, nervous conditions, or skin disorders. Acne and eczema can also be helped with this juice and thereby giving you more beauty.

Eat the tops of asparagus by cooking and juice the stems. When you drink, the juice your urine will have a different smell, which indicates your body is detoxifying.

Avocado Juice

Actually, there is no juice that is made from avocados but is it put in a blender with other foods to create extremely beneficial food. Avocado is considered a complete food because it contains protein, minerals, vitamins, and fatty acids. Avocado has fat in the form of fatty acids – omega 3, omega 6, and omega 9. These fatty acids do not contribute to body fat as many people think, so avocados do not make you fat if you eat them. The fats they have lubricate all your joints and you will find that you will not have joint pain when you eat avocado consistently.

Avocado juice is used for people with malnutrition. The fats in the avocado help to bring the person back slowly and safely to a better nutritional state.

Brain Beet Root Juice Recipe

Beetroot resembles turnips. These roots should not be used in summer since it could disturb your sleep or increase your blood pressure. Use in the winter to keep your body warm and reduce the frequency of colds.

It is an excellent tonic for the nervous system and helps to emulsify and dissolve brain tumors.

Beet root's sweet juice nourishes and enriches the blood. It's helpful in removing mental dementia and healing wounds. It is a **diuretic** and promotes general health and removes toxins from the body.

You can drink this juice daily if you like.

Make 3 to 5 oz. of beetroot

Mix with 12 to 10 oz. of carrot juice

Add 3 to 4 oz. of coconut milk

In this recipe get a combination that is highly alkaline –

potassium, sodium, calcium, magnesium, and iron – and this also contains phosphorus, sulfur, silicon, and chlorine.

Do not drink beet juice alone, it can cause a cleansing reaction, make you dizzy or cause nausea. If you have just started using this juice, start with a few ounces then build up gradually too large amounts.

This juice can be used to build up your red corpuscles.

This juice is a great bodybuilder and helps to clean out your kidneys and gallbladder. The combination of beet, carrot and cucumber juice is also an effective way to clean out your kidneys and gallbladder.

This juice is able to clear the blood of toxin and to help rebuild the liver, kidney, lungs, heart, and brain, which have been all damaged by the addictive behavior.

Pancreas Brussels Sprouts Juice Recipe

You can use Brussels sprouts juice with the following juices

- Carrot
- string bean
- lettuce juices

Start with a little bit of each juice except carrot juice. Use about 6 oz. or carrot juice and add an ounce of each of the other juices. Remember to add the amount to make it drinkable.

This juice will strengthen and regenerate the pancreas for more insulin production. This combination is great if you have diabetes.

If you have cystic fibrosis, then you need to use this juice. Try using one cup in the morning and evening mixed with carrot juice. Also, add them to your vegetable mix.

Cabbage Juice

Cabbage juice is well known for curing duodenum ulcers, but it has a strong taste. Try combining with carrot juice for a more palatable drink. It contains a substance called vitamin U, which is not really a vitamin. It is Vitamin U that gives cabbage juice its power to eliminate or cure stomach or duodenal ulcers. Heating cabbage or cabbage juice will destroy the vitamin U and its ability to relieve ulcers.

Mix it with other juices, such carrot to make it tastier. Drink 2 to 4 oz. of cabbage juice 4 to 5 times per day for up to 10 to 14 days.

Drinking cabbage juice regularly can help you reduce nervousness, fear, depression, headaches, restlessness, and trembling, anxiety, and pessimistic views.

Use cabbage juice, when ill, since it increases the immune system and is a general tonic for the whole body.

Carrot Juice

Carrot juice is the king of juices since it has so many health benefits and can be mixed with other juices to make them more palatable. It rejuvenates the body, produces fresh blood, cleanses the body, produces glowing skin, and provides nutrients for healthy eyes and liver. For those that have a health issue, carrot juice daily is a must to help bring the body back to health.

Its juice helps you maintain the proper balance between alkaline and acid body. Because of its high vitamin A and E, carrot juice is effective in promoting bones and teeth and most importantly the maintenance of healthy body tissues and glandular function.

If you have a low white blood count then carrot juice can bring it up.

You can take carrot juice indefinitely and in any reasonable quantity – 1 to 4 pints a day is ok.

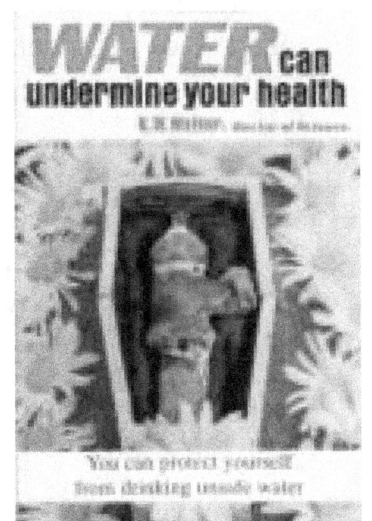

In his book, N.W. Walker, Doctor of Science, Water can undermine your health, Prescott, Norwalk Press, 1974, recounts his experience with carrot juice,

"There was a time when I first started drinking carrot juice that my skin took on an orange-yellow hue. I discovered that this was due to the cleansing of my liver, which happened to be in VERY bad condition at the time. However, after a few months, the discoloration disappeared and my skin was better and clearer than it had ever been. "

If you decide to drink carrot juice daily, there could be a time when you start to feel sick or distressed. Most likely it's not a result of drinking too much juice but more that you have a lot of body toxins to get rid of.

Carrot juice is great for improving your eyesight. If you need to pass an eyesight test and are worried you might not, drink a few glasses of carrot juice daily for a few weeks and then take your test.

Celery Juice

This has a high level of potassium. If you need potassium, then this is the juice to drink. You can add carrot juice to this juice to make it more palatable. Celery juice is also high in sodium and is considered a sodium food. To keep your stomach working like it should it needs a log of organic sodium.

If you frequently feel nervous or agitated, try drinking a combination of celery and carrot juice. This combination is good for restoring the function of degenerating nerve sheathing.

In the case, where you feel like you have an acid body, then celery juice is a must.

1 part carrot juice

¼ part celery juice

You can use more celery juice as you get used to the taste.

Low Blood Cucumber Juice Recipe

Cucumber juice is a great source of manganese and is high in vitamin A. If you have a low blood count then this is the juice for you. Cucumber juice is one of the best diuretics you can use when you need to promote urine. With its high potassium content, it is good for high and low blood pressure.

This juice has also been found to be helpful in skin eruptions.

Mix the following juices together.
- Celery
- Cucumber
- Carrot
- Apple juice – add this juice to make the drink taste better.\

Hardening Of The Arteries Garlic Onion Juice Recipe

Garlic belongs to the onion family. It is recommended not to juice garlic since you can get the liquid form in a two-ounce bottle from Kyolic.

When juicing onion, try to find the Vidalia or Walla Walla onions since they are sweeter.

A dropper of Kyolic garlic

1/4 cup or less of onion juice

Handful of parsley

Handful of spinach or watercress

6 oz. of carrot juice

Start slowly with the use of these juices and experiment with the quantity until you get used to their tastes.

The combination of onion and garlic provide many complex compounds, but they have 3 important minerals – sulfur, potassium, and germanium.

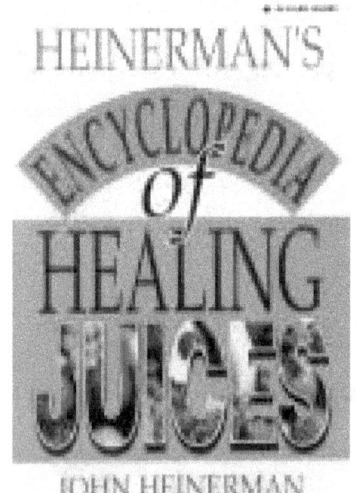

In his book, Heinerman, John, Heinerman's Encyclopedia of Healing Juices, Parker Publishing Company, New York,1994, says it all about garlic and onion,

"The final and most important mineral in garlic and onions is sulfur. Doctors, nutritionists, and health writers don't seem to give much attention to this particular trace element.

I've spent almost a decade studying this tremendously important mineral and have discovered in all of the research surveyed (including my own) that it is the key to preventing hardening of the arteries, cholesterol buildup in the heart, and to stopping drug-resistant forms of bacteria and fungus. When combined with other elements such as potassium and germanium in spices like garlic and onion, a powerful trio of chelating agents are formed which keep the heart and liver free of fatty deposits, the immune defenses alert and active, and the condition of the skin healthy and young."

Green Juices

A green drink can help your pancreas to control sugar blood levels through the production of insulin. It does this by rebuilding the pancreas so that glucagon and insulin are created throughout the day.

A green drink can be used every day. Try to use a green drink at least twice a week.

Using liquid chlorophyll is great if you don't have a green drink.

1 – 2 oz. of liquid chlorophyll

6 oz. of distilled water

The juice of 1/2 lemon or lime

This can be drunk every day first thing in the morning.

Blue Green Manna is another powder you can use. It is high in chlorophyll and enzymes in the chlorophyll. This Manna is great for regulating the pancreas. You can check out this site for capsules.

Blue Green Manna – 1 tablespoon

6 oz. of distilled water

2 oz. of pineapple, apple, or grape juice

You can add a couple of ounces of fresh pineapple, apple, and grape juice to make it more palatable. Adding a pinch of honey is another way to take a green drink.

For kids, you can add the green drink or green manna into jello.

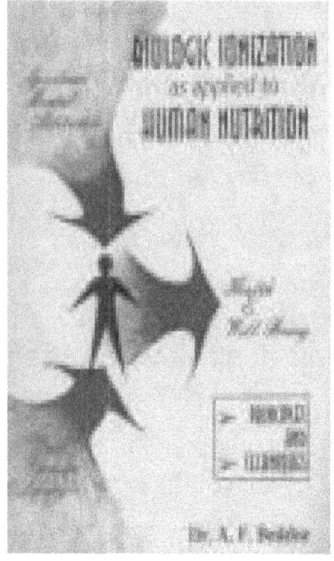

In his book, Dr. Beddoe, A.F., Biologic Ionization as applied to Human Nutrition, S & J Unlimited, Washington, 1994, gives you a recipe for a fresh green drink that you can prepare with a blender,

"Take 2 cups of your favorite juice and place it in a good quality high-speed blender. Add to it this large handful of greens chosen from the list the follows this paragraph. The amount will vary according to the type of blender used. . . Add as much as can be chopped and blended thoroughly and comfortably, until all greens have well blended for a period of time (3 to 4 minutes) turn of the blender and pour the mixture through a kitchen strainer to remove the pulp. The juice that is left is the green drink."

Use any of the following green leaves:

Bean, dandelion, nasturtium leaves, parsley, wheatgrass, pea pods, romaine lettuce, spinach, beet, carrot tops, celery stalk tops, kale, or any other dark green leaves.

The more chlorophyll you can drink and get into your body the better. Chlorophyll is one of the compounds that green drinks give you. Chlorophyll will slowly chelate, tie up and remove toxic heavy metals out of your body. It gives you great antibacterial and antiviral protection. And it gives you good oxygenation for your cells. And, then it is one of the best blood cleansers and rejuvenators. It helps to build your blood, giving you the youth factors you need to stay young.

Kale and Collard Juices

Kale is very high in alkaline minerals like calcium and in vitamin A. You can mix kale juice with carrot or pineapple juice. Drinking kale or collard juices will help you absorb more calcium that you do when you drink milk.

Hemorrhoid Mustard Greens Juice Recipe

Pure mustard greens juice has an irritating effect on the gastrointestinal tract and the kidney. By combining this juice with carrot, spinach and turnip juice, you will get relief for your hemorrhoids.

Mustard greens have a high level of oxalic acid and should never be eaten cooked. When cooked, the oxalic acid is turned from organic oxalic acid, a natural nutrient your body can use, to an inorganic oxalic acid that your body cannot use. Inorganic oxalic acid is destructive in your body since it causes the formation of kidney oxalic crystal – kidney stones.

Urinary Parsley Juice Tonic

Parsley juice should never be taken alone, but a small amount, one to two oz., should be mixed with other vegetable juice like,

- Parsley a small handful
- Carrot
- Spinach

You can also mix it with lime and orange juice to get a different taste. It helps in keeping your blood vessels functioning normal. It has a tonic effect on the urinary system by removing urinary problems like bladder pain and swelling. It is also useful in kidney diseases.

It is also useful in relieving cramps associated with menstrual irregularities. But it has to be used a little more concentrated with the above juices mentioned.

Skin Blemish Potato Juice Recipe

The combination of eating meat and cooked potatoes has the effect of intensifying the solanine poison, an alkaloid, of the potato. Green potatoes have a higher concentration of this poison.

- Potato juice

- Carrot juice

The juice of potatoes is quite digestible and has proven to be helpful in clearing up skin blemishes. Combine it with carrot juice to get a better tasting juice.

If you have stomach problems, sensitive nerves, gout, or sciatica, then create this juice with Potato, carrots, beet, and cucumber juice.

Blood Purifier Radish Juice Recipe

At least 1/3 of radish content is potassium and 1/3 is sodium. The radish is also high in iron and magnesium.

It's great for eyesight, nerve soother, and to eliminate intestinal worms. It is useful for removing kidney and gall-bladder stones. It is also useful to rejuvenate and rebuild muscles.

The juice can be used to massage into wrinkles to minimize them.

Radish juice has a pungent taste and should never be drunk alone. It is best to use this mixture, radish, carrots, tomatoes, lemon.

In Russian research, they discovered that the sulfur in red radishes was able to keep the production of the thyroid's thyroxine and calcitonin in balance. All that is needed is eating a few radishes a day or drinking a little radish juice mixed with other juices – carrot, tomato, or celery.

General Spinach Juice Tonic

Spinach juice should be used by anyone with anemia because of its high iron content. It is also useful in the entire gastrointestinal tract and especially useful for constipation and nervous disorders. Use Spinach juice as a general or nerve tonic. Spinach and Cabbage juice are good for neuralgia, a pain that runs along a damaged nerve.

If you drink pure spinach juice in the morning, it will remove chronic constipation and toxic matter from the colon.

If you're pregnant, this juice will help you eliminate low iron deficiency. It will help you improve your and your baby's health. Use it with other juices especially carrot

- Spinach 2oz.
- Carrot 6 oz.
- Celery a small amount of this juice
- Cucumber a small amount of this juice

Spinach is also high in organic oxalic acid and should not be eaten cooked. Eat it raw or juiced to get the natural oxalic acid that your body needs.

Blood Tomato Juice Recipe

Tomato juice is to be used in raw form. It is a blood purifier and stimulates the blood circulation. It cleanses your body of toxins and is a worm killer. Tomatoes help keep your blood alkaline, reduce body acidity, resist diseases, cure liver, and spleen disorders, fights cardiovascular disease, and also remove chronic fever.

Use tomato juice, when you have a cold or flu. Those that have diabetes or prone to nervous conditions should drink tomato juice regularly.

- Tomato 6 oz.
- Carrots 2 oz.
- 1/2 lemon juice

In cooked form, citric, malic, and oxalic acids become inorganic compounds and have a detrimental effect on your body.

When this raw juice is drunk with starches or sugar, it acts as an acid food otherwise the body sees it as an alkaline food.

10: Special Tonics That Block Aging & Promote Youth

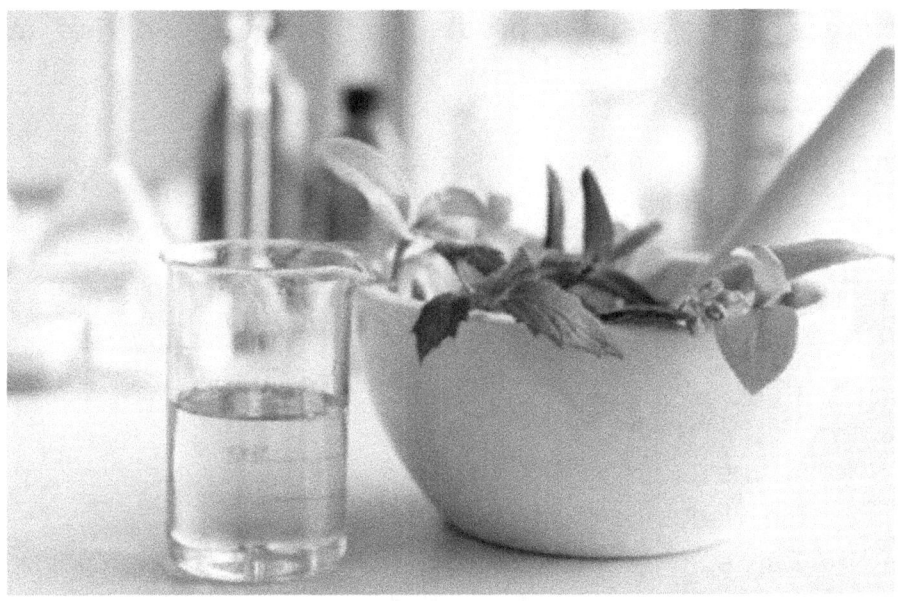

In this chapter, you will find some special tonics that are designed for a specific illness. Use these tonics even though you might not identify with these illnesses. The formulations are designed to provide you with nutrients that target specific parts of the body. But because these are tonics they not only help a target area but also help to normalize many of your other body functions.

Use these tonics, when you have a slight indication of the illness targeted. The reason for this is you want to make sure you have the best health because this is where your youthful appearance will come from an energy that is associated with youth.

These tonics will increase your body's tone and give you increase energy and strength. In addition, they provide the nutrients that you need to regenerate cells, tissue, and organs and thus providing you with anti-aging benefits.

Here are the main ingredients that you will find in these tonics.

- Wheat germ oil
- Brewer's yeast
- Raw wheat germ
- Soya powder
- Pressed wheat germ oil
- Apple cider vinegar
- Whey powder
- Soybean oil
- Unsweetened gelatin powder
- Raw sunflower seeds grounded
- Raw sesame seeds grounded
- Wheat germ flakes

When you prepare these tonics, keep close to the recipes. What you can do is add something to these recipes to make them more palatable.

Digestive Tonic

Here is a tonic you can mix to help you normalize your digestion. This will neutralize excess acid and dilute stomach gas. Juice the following and drink 1 hour before your 3 meals.

- 3 cucumbers
- 1 celery bunch
- Juice of half a lemon
- A bunch of dark green lettuce

Skin Tonic

- Mix the following juices,
- One part berry juice
- One part apricot juice
- A bit of honey

This tonic will help to moisturize your skin and lubricate skin cells and tissue. It will give your skin a healthy glow.

Mix the following juices,
- One part orange juice
- One part grapefruit juice
- One whole lemon juice

Go heavy on the lemon juice. This drink provides a bundle of vitamin C and other antioxidant nutrients. With its abundant minerals, it will help move your body towards alkalinity. This tonic promotes skin health, skin rejuvenation, skin cell growth, improves skin flaking, and improves skin metabolism.

This tonic will rejuvenate your skin and improve your health at the same time. This is a beauty tonic.

- Juice fresh 3 to 4 oranges

- Juice a few slices of pineapple
- 1 tsp. brewer's yeast
- 4 tbs. of raw wheat germ
- 1 tbs. of soya powder
- 1 banana
- Honey to taste
- 1 tsp. of blackstrap molasses
- 1 teaspoon of whey powder
- 4 slices of fresh apricots or organic dry

Prepare this in the morning for breakfast or as a midmorning snack. It's the liquid of the juices and tonics that give your skin the water and nutrients it needs to give you beauty.

Hair Growing Tonic

Here is a tonic that gives you the vitamin E that you need to nourish the hair bulb to stimulate hair growth. Your body needs an oversupply of nutrients to keep your hair strong and growing. Your body uses the nutrients you supply it and if it has extra nutrients your hair will be nourished.

- ¼ cup cold pressed wheat germ oil
- ¼ cup soybean oil
- 4 tablespoons of apple cider vinegar
- 4 tablespoons of apple juice
- ½ cup of fresh vegetable oil – olive oil or coconut oil, etc.

Completely mix the oils and drink slowly. Drink this every day to get the vitamin E that will bring oxygen to your scalp.

Hair growth via thyroid

Hair grow is also controlled by your cell metabolism. If you have hypothyroidism, this will reduce your hair beauty and hair growth. The following tonic will normalize your thyroid function and improve your hair health.

- 1/2 cup unsweetened gelatin powder
- 2 tablespoons brewer's yeast
- 1/2 to 1 cup freshly squeezed orange juice

Drink this juice 3 times a day. To improve the effectiveness of this hair tonic, eliminate the use of sugar in soft drinks and foods. When you do this, you maximize the power of this hair tonic.

Drinking juices and tonics will help your hair grow and look healthy because liquids quickly get into your bloodstream and flow to your scalp to feed your hair.

Youth Beauty Tonic

It's the enzymes that are king in the juices and tonics that you drink, which can help you maintain your youth. They do this by being active in 1000's of chemical reactions that occur in your body that prevent degradation of all body elements. This is one of the main reasons that many people lose their beauty and youth. They don't eat enough fresh fruits and vegetables that packed with digestive enzymes.

Here is a tonic that is packed with enzymes.

- 1/2 cup of raw sunflower seeds grounded
- 1/2 cup of raw sesame seeds grounded
- 1 cup of distilled water
- 2 tsp. of honey
- A pinch of sea salt
- 1/2 tsp. of soy milk powder

The following enzyme anti-aging tonic is packed with nutrients that will revive and regenerate your body so that you feel and look young.

- 6 tbs. cold-pressed wheat germ oil
- 1/2 cup freshly squeezed carrot juice
- 1/2 cup freshly squeezed lettuce juice
- 1/2 cup freshly squeezed cucumber juice
- 2 tbs. apple cider vinegar

Drink this tonic after lunch every day.

Arthritis Tonic

If you have slight pain in your joints, now would be a good time to take care of this issue before it gets worse and takes away your youth.

Mix the following,

- 6 tbs. of wheat germ
- 3/4 cup of fresh orange juice
- 1/4 cup of fresh grapefruit juice

Drink this mixture three times a day. This tonic will help circulate your blood better to your leg and to reduce arthritic pain. It helps to reduce restless legs.

Bioflavonoid arthritic tonic

Drink one glass of this tonic to reduce arthritic pain every day.

- ½ cup freshly squeezed orange juice
- ½ cup freshly squeezed grape juice
- 1 tbs. lemon juice
- 2 tbs. dark organic honey

Cartilage Tonic

Its the vitamin C that provides the nutrient for cartilage, collagen, connective tissue, bones, muscles, and vascular tissues. Here's how to get the power to strengthen your bone and tissue structure.

- 1/2 cup grapefruit juice
- 1/4 cup orange juice
- 1/4 cup apricot juice
- 2 tbs. rose hips powder
- The juice of 1/2 lemon

Drink this tonic one hour before all three meals.

Blood Circulation Tonic

With this tonic, you will feel the power of youth returning. This drink will bring color back to your face and improve your appearance. It is packed with potassium and iron.

- 1/2 cup of freshly squeezed grape juice
- 1/2 cup of raisin juice
- 1 tbs. of lemon juice
- 1 tsp. apple cider vinegar

Drink this tonic two times a day.

Mineral Tonic

Minerals are used throughout your body for building all parts of it. In addition, they are the main elements that reduce the acid produced in your body. It is the unneutralized body acids that diminish your youth and beauty.

Mix and drink this tonic every day.

- One part carrot juice
- One part celery juice
- One part radish juice
- 2 tbs. of onion juice

Another mineral tonic

- 1/2 cup of raisin juice
- 1/2 cup of apricot juice
- 1 tbs. of lemon juice
Drink this tonic twice a day.

Potassium Mineral tonic

Here is another powerful mineral tonic that will provide nutrients for the whole body. It is a tonic packed with potassium and other minerals and vitamins.

Boil distilled water and turn off heat

In a bowl put any of the following dried fruits together – peaches, apricots, raisins, prunes, and pears.

Pour hot water into the bowl and cover

Let bowl with fruits sit overnight

In the morning drink one cup of this juice

Eat fruit as a breakfast

This tonic will help make you regular, neutralize body acid, activate kidney and detoxify the body, provide iron for blood creating hemoglobin, and provide B vitamins.

Beauty mineral tonic

This tonic will provide your skin, nails, and cells with the nutrients it needs to be healthy.

Mix together the following in equal portions.

Cranberry, pineapple, berry juice and then add a tbs. of lemon juice.

Anemia Iron Tonic

Here is a tonic that you can use to build up your iron body stores. If you feel tired, you can boost your hemoglobin production to provide more oxygen to your cells with this tonic.

- 3 tablespoons of unflavored gelatin powder
- Two tablespoons of desiccated liver powder
- 1 cup of tomato juice
- A splash of lemon juice
- Drink one glass an hour before meals.

Another Iron Tonic

Equal parts of celery and carrot juice
Add one part parsley or just a small handful. Parsley is a powerful tasting herb and should not be drunk alone. Add parsley to these juices until you can accept the taste.

Protein Power Tonic

- 3 Tbs. of unflavored gelatin powder
- 1 whole banana
- 1 cup of soy milk, rice dream, or almond milk

Blend these ingredients and drink three glasses a day. This protein tonic will improve blood health, heal kidneys, control weight, repair the body, and feeds all parts of the body.

Insomnia Sleep Tonic

These are a few sleep tonics you can use if you don't get enough sleep. Getting enough sleep will ensure that you have plenty of day energy and that you live a longer life.

- 1 tbs. of brewer's yeast powder
- 1 tbs. of soybean powder or whey or goat whey powder
- 1 tbs. of wheat germ flakes
- 1 tbs. of sunflower seed oil
- Place in a blender and add distilled water

Drink this tonic about an hour before bedtime.

- Here is a **sleep tonic** that will provide you with calcium to relax you and prepare you for bedtime.
- 1 cup milk, skim or whole
- 2 tbs. rice polish
- 1 tablespoon natural honey
- 1 tbs. powdered skim milk
- 1 tsp. carob powder

Combine all ingredients into a blender and blend for a good minute or two. To add more sleeping power into this tonic, add a banana to the blender.

A **simple sleep tonic**, in case you don't have many ingredients, is to use the following.

- 2 whole bananas

- 1 cup of skim or soy milk
- 2 tbs. of honey

Blend everything in a blender, then drink 1 hour before bedtime.

Fatigue Tonic

- 1/2 cup prune juice
- 1/2 cup orange juice
- 1/8 cup grapefruit juice

Drink this tonic around 30 minutes after your 3 meals. This tonic helps cleanse your kidney, improves blood circulation and stimulates metabolism.

Artery Cleansing Tonic

- 1 tablespoon of lecithin granules or powder
- 1 glass of tomato juice
- 1 tablespoon of brewer's yeast
- Mix them in a blender for a minute
-

Drink three glasses each day before meals.

Lecithin has a cleansing action on the artery walls and is capable of reducing fat globules into tiny droplets to make fats more absorbable in the small intestine. Use Lecithin wherever you can like in salads, soups, and smoothies.

Allergy Lemon Cayenne Tonic

Here is a tonic that will soothe a sore throat and is

Good for combating a cold.

- 3/4 cup freshly squeezed lemon juice
- ¼ cup honey
- 1 cup purified water
- 1/4 to 1/2 teaspoon cayenne

After you mix everything thoroughly, you can drink this hot or cold. This will give you a good feeling. This tonic is only for children older than 6 years and adults.

General Body Tonic

Combine coconut juice and carrot juice in equal amounts. If you buy coconuts, you can get the juice that is in the center of the coconut, when you open it.

This tonic is good for colitis, stomach issues, liver complaints, nervous exhaustion, and constipation. It is a good tasting tonic.

11: Basic Principle Of Smoothies That Give Health

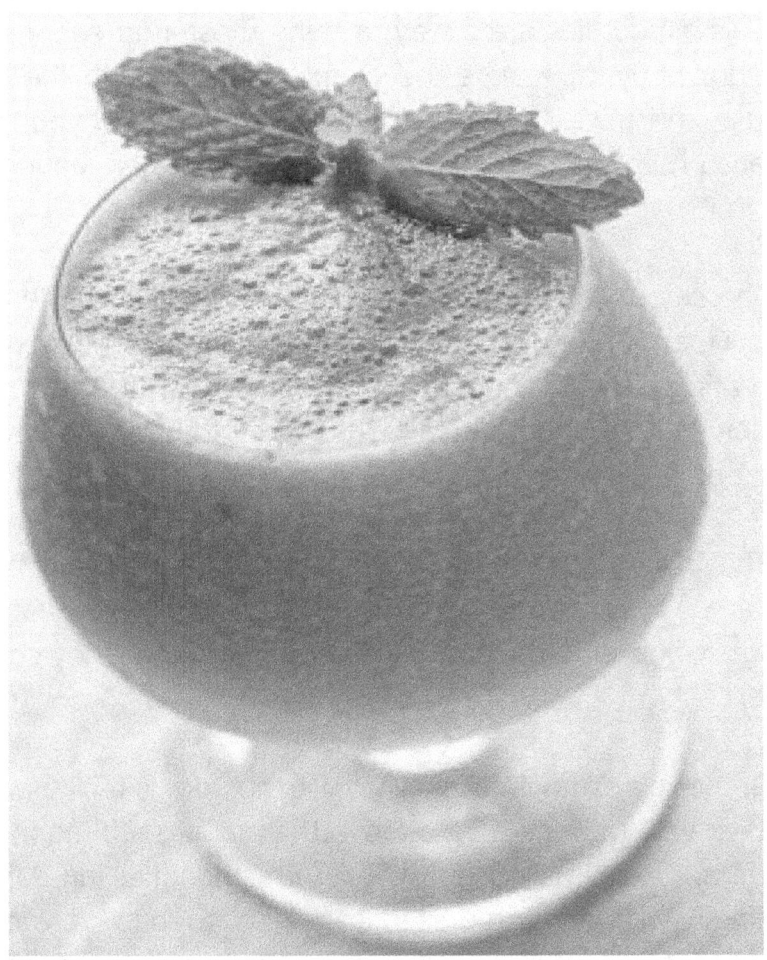

Fruits Smoothies That Keep You Youthful

Fruit smoothies provide you with a different way to eat fruits and drink their juices. Smoothies mixed with other power ingredients and nutrients can serve to give you better health. Smoothies can be used to build, cleanse, and heal your body. The result is that they give you the most beauty you can achieve.

In cases where you are depleted of various vitamins and minerals, smoothies are a way to bring these nutrients quickly into your body. Because the blender grinds down the fruits you use and mixes them with any juices you use, your body will absorb this mixture much faster than when eating the solid fruit.

The smoothies listed here also provide you with plenty of fiber. Fiber is one of the main foods you want to increase in your eating plan. It is fiber that your body needs every day to function well. Without at least 30 grams of fiber each day you cannot be healthy.

This is why smoothies have a special place in your health program. They can be used every day to help you eat fruit with their fiber and the special healing juices that they contain inside.

Drink your smoothie slowly. Do not drink it like water. The best way to drink it is to move the mixture around in your mouth so saliva is mixed with the smoothie ingredients. Drinking a smoothie too fast can lead to gas (air in the smoothie) to form in the stomach and intestine, which can cause some discomfort.

Once your smoothie is made, drink it within a few minutes. The smoothie ingredients will start to oxidize and decay quickly as it has air mixed in from the blending process.

If you fill a thermos to the top, you can use the smoothie for later, but it is always best to add a teaspoon or more of powdered vitamin C to act as a preservative.

Using fresh fruit and if possible fresh juices will provide you with a mixture that will add more minerals to your body and thereby making your body's pH more alkaline.

In her book, The Big Book of Juices and Smoothies, 2003, Natalie Savona, gives some hints on storing your smoothie.

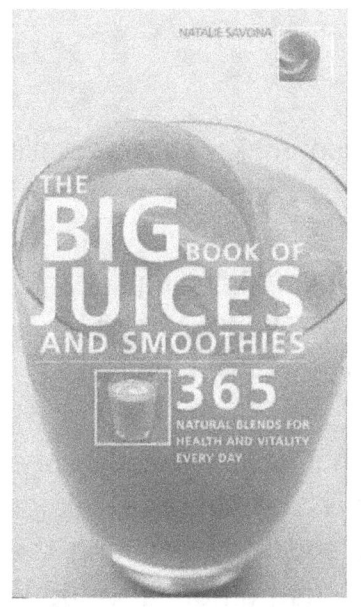

"There really is no such thing as storing a juice or smoothie – you can't beat drinking them the moment you've made them. However, you may like to take them out to work or on a picnic. In that case, the best way to store them is to put a teaspoon of vitamin C powder or a squeeze of lemon juice in the bottom of the jug attached to the juicer. The vitamin C acts as an antioxidant, preventing the juice from turning brown. The same goes for smoothies. Also keep the drinks covered and cool – in a sealed container in the refrigerator, or in a thermos flask"

Smoothie Base

Here is how you build a smoothie that can give many health benefits. The smoothie base is a liquid slurry that can be used to add more ingredients.

The liquid base can be made from various fresh juices or rice, oat, or almond milk. Stay away from milk since milk creates mucus along the gastrointestinal lining. Choose and mix any of the following liquid and pour them into a blender.

Juices – apple, pineapple, orange, tangerine, lemon
Milk – rice dream, oat milk, almond milk. Use a combination of 40% rice dream, 40% almond milk, and 20% apple juice or you can use the combinations you like.

Sesame Milk

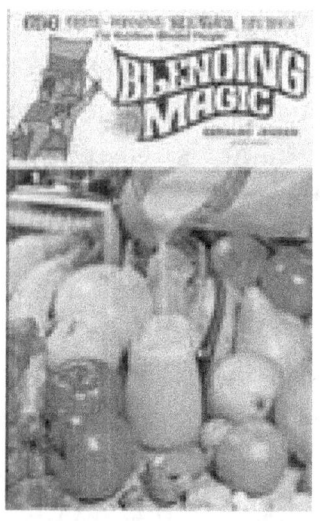

You can also make sesame milk and use this in your smoothies.

In his book, Blending Magic, Bernard Jensen, Nutritionist, has a really nice recipe for sesame milk.

"I believe that sesame seed is one of our best. It is a wonderful drink for gaining weight and for lubricating the intestinal tract. Its nutritional value is beyond compare, as it is high in protein and minerals. This is the seed that is used as a basic food in Arabia and East India."

Blend for 1- 1 1/2 minutes to make smooth,

- 2 cups of distilled water
- 1/4 cup of Sesame Seed, run these seeds through a coffee grinder to make a powder.

- 2 Tablespoons Soy Milk Powder

In place of 2 cups of distilled water, you can use 1 cup of water and 1 cup of low-fat rice dream. If you use goat whey powder, this will add to the mineral power of this drink.

Banana Base

Next, use bananas your smoothies. This gives the liquid a bit more thickness. Also bananas are high in potassium and other minerals. Use bananas that are not overripe since they have too much sugar. Do not use under-ripe bananas, since they will create acid in your body, as will all other fruits that are not ripe and ready to eat.

Main Ingredients

Next, choose a fruit that will be the main ingredient so you can say you are making a strawberry smoothie or a blueberry smoothie. If you have fresh organic fruit, then this is the best way to create your smoothie. What you can do is freeze fruits during its season, so you can have some of this fruit a bit longer than its seasonal run. Choose from fruits that are in season.

- Avocado
- Cantaloupe, watermelon
- Peach, mango, papaya, guava
- Pineapple, apricots, apples
- Strawberries, blueberries, raspberries
- Figs
- Dried prunes, peaches, apricots, fig

More Nutrients to Add

Once you have your basic smoothie, you can add other nutrients that will provide you with additional fiber, oil, vitamins, minerals, and many other nutrients.

Here is a short list of some of the ingredients you can add to your smoothies. Add only 2-3 other ingredients so the tastes don't get too complex or unusual. But it's up to you what you add to your smoothie. The more you add to it the more nutritional power it will have to make or keep you beautiful and healthy.

- Almonds
- Beet Juice powder
- Blackstrap molasses
- Capra mineral whey
- Chia Seeds
- ROI water Ice cubes
- Edible dairy whey
- Fig Juice syrup
- Flaxseed and flaxseed oil
- Honey, rice syrup
- Lecithin granules
- Powder vitamin C
- Raisins
- Rice or oat bran
- Sesame seeds
- Sunflower seeds, pumpkin seeds

Wheat germ

Ruby Red is a powder which contains 35 fruit powders. This gives your smoothie a boost of vitamins, minerals, probiotics, antioxidants, phytonutrients, and digestive enzymes. It's an excellent blend to use giving your smoothie a tremendous nutritional boost.

Make sure you add a tablespoon or more of lecithin granules. This helps to keep your arteries clean and blood thinner. Lecithin also has Choline which helps to create acetylcholine a neurotransmitter for your brain. Lecithin is used in used in every cell of your body and is a necessary nutrient.

You can add bran and whole seeds into the blender and it will break them up if it is a high-speed blender. It is best to put seeds or bran into a coffee grinder to create a powder.

Smoothie Recipes

So, here are a few smoothie recipes you can blend. In this recipes, you can leave out the rice dream and replace it with the fresh juice listed in the recipe.

- Apple Smoothie
- Apricot Smoothie

- Peach-Rice Dream Smoothie
- Pineapple Smoothie
- Strawberry Smoothie

- Sweet-Yams-Banana Smoothie
- Papaya Smoothie
- Prune and Apple Juice Blend
- High Fiber Breakfast Smoothie
- Papaya Smoothie

Apple Smoothie

Mix in the blender the following.

- 1-2 small apples cut into wedges
- 1 banana
- 1 cup 50:50 rice dream: almond milk
- ¼ cup or less of raisins soaked overnight
- 1-teaspoon honey
- 1-2 cubes of ice
- 1-teaspoon lecithin granules
- 2 teaspoons flaxseed oil

Start by mixing the banana and the liquids. Then add slices of apples to get the consistency you like.

Apricot Smoothie

- One cup of fresh apricots or dried apricots that was soaked overnight
- Juice of 1/2 a lemon
- Two oz. of prune juice
- One teaspoon or more of oat ban
- One teaspoon of mineral whey
- Add a slight amount of distilled water to make the consistency to your liking.

Peach-Rice Dream Smoothie

Mix in the blender:

- 2 fresh peaches with peel
- 1-cup rice dream
- 1/2 banana
- 1-teaspoon sesame seeds grounded
- 1-teaspoon sunflower seed grounded
- 1-teaspoon lecithin granules
- 2 teaspoons flaxseed oil

Pineapple Smoothie

Mix the following in a blender.

- 1-2 cups of fresh pineapples
- 1/2 cups apple slices
- 3/4 cup fresh apple juice
- 1 banana
- 1-teaspoon lecithin
- 1-teaspoon flax seeds grounded
- 2 teaspoons bran (wheat, oat or rice) grounded

Strawberry Smoothie

Mix in a blender the following ingredients.

- 1 banana
- 1-teaspoon of lecithin granules
- 1-teaspoon of any type of bran grounded
- 1 cup or less of almond milk

Now add strawberries one by one with the blender on until you get the consistency you like.

Now in a coffee grinder, grind the following and add them to the blended strawberry mix:

- 1-teaspoon flax seeds
- 1 or 2 teaspoon sunflower seeds
- 1-teaspoon sesame seeds

Sweet-Yam-Banana Smoothie

Mix the following together.

- 1-2 cups of baked yams or sweet potatoes
- 1 small banana
- 1-teaspoon honey or maple syrup
- 1 cup of rice dream or apple juice (more or less as needed)
- 1-teaspoon lecithin granules
- 1-teaspoon flax seed oil

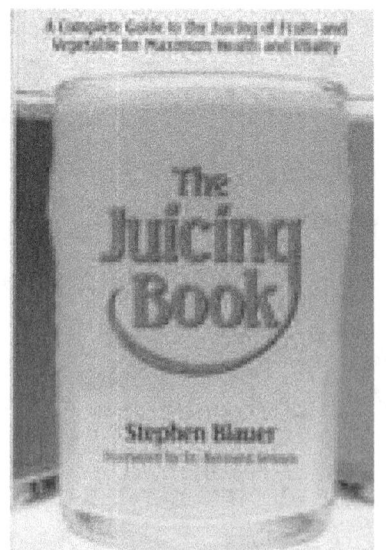

- 2 teaspoons of bran you like

You can make the consistency to be pudding-like and pour into small cups, place in the refrigerator to cool and then serve.

Papaya Smoothie

In his book, The Juicing Book, 1989, Stephen Blauer lists a papaya smoothie.

"8 dried apricot halves

1 large apple

1/2   papaya,   peeled   and   pitted
Soak Apricots overnight in one-cup water. Discard soak water
before juicing. Wash apple. Juice apple and papaya.
Combine apricots with apple and papaya juice. Blend for one
minute on medium speed."

To improve this smoothie, for relieving constipation, add a
couple of slices of apple and papaya into the blender to
provide some fiber. Then add some lecithin, ground up flax
seeds.

Soaking Dried Fruits

To use dried fruit in your smoothies, you need to soak
them. Why soak them?

Soaking them in hot water kills any insects, parasite and
other pathogens on the fruit. Soaking makes the fruit more
digestible and available for absorption

Un-soaked fruit can cause gas to form in the stomach
since it takes more time for the digestive juices to penetrate
them and dissolve them.

Soaking them prevents the fruit from passing out the
rectum undigested. Undigested fruit can petrify in your colon
when you have constipation.

Here's how to soak your dried fruit.

Twelve hours before or the night before using the fruit, place the fruit in a glass pot and cover slightly with distilled water.

Heat the water just too where it starts to boil and pull the pot off the stove. Cover and let sit overnight

The next morning used the soaked fruit in the blender.

Soak all dried fruits in this manner, including raisins. When using dried apricots, use only naturally dried apricots without sulfur. These don't look nice and colorful. They look dark and wrinkled but they are healthier.

Prune and Apple Juice Blend

Rinse prunes in distilled water to remove any dirt or contamination. Soak 3/4 cup or more of prunes overnight. Just slightly cover the prunes with distilled water. In the morning, blend prunes with its water and one cup of apple juice. Add a couple slices of apple with its peel. Squeeze 1/2 lemon and blend again.

Add more apple juice to get the consistency you like.

This makes a great morning drink to get your bowel moving later in the morning.

High Fiber Breakfast Smoothie

Here's a drink you can prepare in the morning and can serve as breakfast.

In a blender add,

- One half a banana that is not overripe
- One half an apple
- A few strawberries, fresh or frozen
- ¾ cup or so of rice dream, almond milk, or organic soymilk
- one rounded teaspoon of each bran - wheat, rice, and oat
- one tablespoon of lecithin granules
- one teaspoon of flaxseed oil

The bran will help you bulk up your stool.

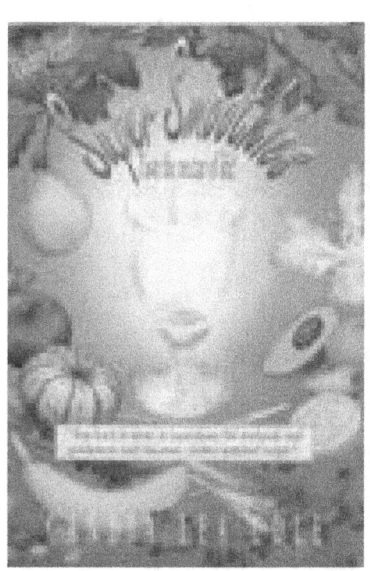

One of the best books on making smoothies is called Super Smoothies, by Candia Lea Cole. The ingredients in her book are good for helping clear constipation. By adding a few more ingredients, as listed above under "More Nutrients to Add", to these smoothies, it will help to create super smoothies for clearing constipation. Most of her smoothies use those fruits and vegetables that help constipation

Mango Cool Smoothie

Combine the following in a blender:

- One peeled and cored mango
- 1/4 to 1/2 cup of orange juice
- 1/2 banana

- a few ice cubes to give it some consistency
- teaspoon of flaxseed oil
- teaspoon to tablespoon of oat bran grounded
- teaspoon of sesame seeds grounded

Papaya Smoothie

Mix in a blender:
- One cupful of papaya
- 1/2 banana
- Juice of one lime or lemon
- Add apple juice to get the consistency you like
- One teaspoon of flaxseed oil
- One teaspoon of goat mineral whey
- One tablespoon of edible dairy whey

Now you have various ingredients that are good for adding more vitamins, minerals, and nutrients to make your body more alkaline.

In addition, these smoothies will help to detoxify your body when used in the first body cycle from 4 am to noon time. You can make your combination according to your taste and enjoyment.

You can make many other smoothies by replacing the fruits listed in the smoothies with the fruits that you like or that are available at your store or farmers market. If you have organic fruit, try using them without peeling them.

12: When To Drink Your Juices

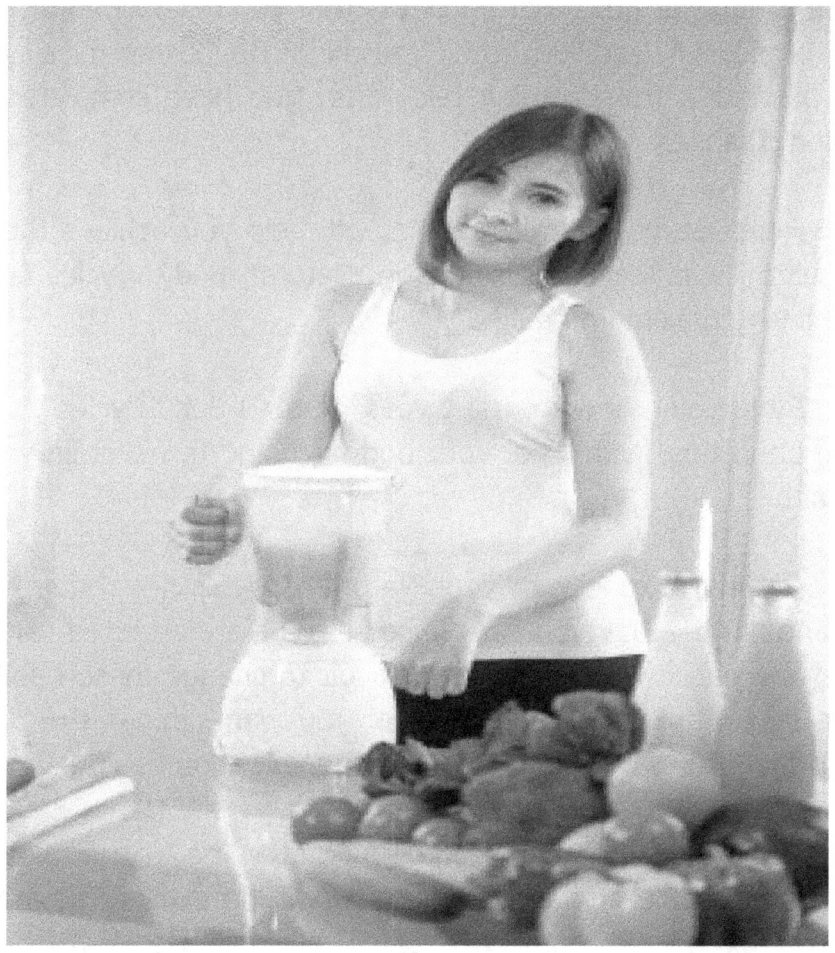

Body Cycle 1

Now that you have completed your body cleanse, here is a way to eat so that you allow your body to keep cleansing itself using its natural body cycle.

Natural Body Cycles

Most of you are looking for ways to improve your health, lose weight, or get rid of an illness that you have. If you have acid reflux or heartburn, then you might be looking for a way to prevent it from coming back after you have completed a colon cleanse.

Here's some information that will help you achieve these results. It is called "Using the Natural Body Cycles" for achieving maximum health.

By learning how to assist your "Natural Body Cycles", you will be in tune with what your body is doing to maintain your health.

Getting in tune with your Natural Body Cycles requires a change in the way you eat. Since all of us are addicted to the way we eat, it is, sometimes, difficult to change these habits. But if you are serious about what you want, this is the best information I have found that will give you good health.

Using this method to gain better health, you will experience side effects because you will be eliminating more body toxins and body wastes. The side effects may be headaches, stomach upsets, body pain, or similar types of symptoms. These conditions will not last and will disappear as you get rid of more toxins. So if you experience these side effects, don't let them stop you from moving forward on this eating pattern.

Here are the 3 natural body cycles:

Cycle 1 time period: 4 a.m. to 12 noon

This cycle is the time where your body is eliminating toxins, acids, wastes, and derby by urine, bowel movements, and other secretions.

Cycle 2 time period: 12 noon to 8 p.m.

This is the time when your body should be taking in food and digesting

Cycle 3 time period: 8 p.m. to 4 a.m.

This is the time your body is absorbing and using the food you have eaten during the 12 noon to 8 p.m. period.

Here's how to use cycle 1:

During the elimination cycle, 4 a.m. to 12 noon, eat and drink only fruits and their juices or drink vegetable juices. For breakfast eat a bowl of fruit or have a fruit smoothie made with apple juice and fruits in season.

Before noontime, eat fruits as a snack. Forty-five minutes before noon eat your last fruit. You can eat and drink all the fruits and juices you want up to noontime.

Bananas, oranges, apricots, strawberries, melon, watermelons, apples, peaches, nectarines, and so on.

Eat all melons together and not with other fruit and wait 1/2 hour before eating other fruit. Melons require their specific enzymes to be digested in the stomach so other fruit eaten with melons will just sit in your stomach waiting to be digested. (Not a good idea, I will tell you why in the next newsletter.)

By eating in this way you are assisting your body's elimination cycle. This helps your body to eliminate toxins and acids from your body and blood. It is these toxins and acids that make you sick and overweight.

Eating solid food for breakfast – eggs potatoes, rice, meat, cereal, milk, and so on - interfere with your body's elimination cycle and eventually leads to sickness and excess weight. It takes over 3 hours to digest heavy and solid food. The food you should be eating, in the morning, should digest quickly to help remove toxins, acids, and waste from your body.

Heavy food slows down the elimination of toxins from your body and this causes more toxins to remain in the body to get stored as fat and acids. Acids are the main cause of most illnesses and so you want to have an alkaline body. Fruits and vegetables give you an alkaline body.

It takes a ½ hour or so to digest fruit and fruit juices. Because of this, they help to cleanse your body of waste. Fruits are 70% water just like your body.

So if you are not already having fruit and fruit juices for breakfast and snacks, start slowing changing your habits if you want to lose weight and feel better.

Now, one other thing, don't eat fruits and juices with your lunch or dinner meals.

13: Natural Body Cycle 2

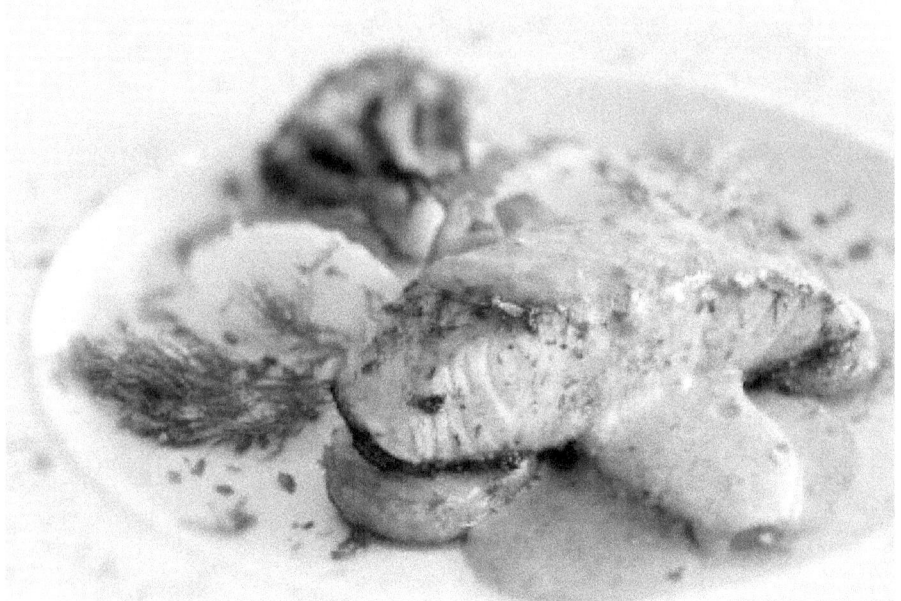

Again these cycles are:

Cycle 1 time period: 4 a.m. to 12 noon

    This cycle is the time where your body is eliminating toxins, acids, wastes, and derby by urine, bowel movements, sweat, mucus, and other secretions.

Cycle 2 time period: 12 noon to 8 p.m.

    This is the time when your body should be taking in food and digesting

Cycle 3 time period: 8 p.m. to 4 a.m.

Let's now discuss Cycle 2 time period: 12 noon to 8 p.m.

During this period is time to eat solid food. What you eat has to be in alignment with what your stomach can do.

Here's how your stomach works. In general, it can only digest one solid food at a time.

Solid food is one that does not contain 70% water, as fruits and vegetables do, and whose water has been eliminated by heat or other food processes, in other words, cooked. Your stomach can only work on one solid food at a time, so your lunch and dinner should only have one solid food. Lunch can consist of chicken and a green salad, fish and a green salad, tuna and a green salad, shrimp and a green salad, beef and a green salad.

Mixing a protein meal with carbohydrates is giving the stomach two solid foods at the same time, which require different concentrations of digestive juices.

Giving the stomach more than it can handle interrupts the elimination cycle 1 and reduces the energy that you need for the elimination cycle.

Any eating habit that disrupts cycle 2, the eating and digestion cycle, affects the other cycles. Here's how you can help your body's cycle 2 to be more effective.

Eat only one solid food with vegetables during lunch or dinner. Lunch can be one meat or seafood with a fresh vegetable salad.

Limit the amount of water you drink during your eating.

Excess water will dilute your digestive acids and slow down the digestion of your food.

Eliminate drinking any sodas, coffee, tea or other drinks during your meals. If you need to clear your dry throat use a little water, which is room temperature. Cold liquids will slow down your digestive processes.

Eating meals with more than one solid food such as meat and potatoes, chicken and rice, fish and rice, chicken and noodles, eggs and toast, cheese and bread will diminish the energy you need during the elimination cycle 1.

It is permissible to eat beef and chicken at the same time but not chicken and eggs or beef and nut or chicken and beans. Eat the same type of protein at the same time but do not mix different proteins.

It's ok to eat different types of carbohydrates at the same time, with a salad, but not with protein, since carbohydrates digest easier than protein.

Eating a protein and a carbohydrate at the same time sets the stage for severe illness later in life. A protein requires acid for digestion and a carbohydrate requires alkaline juices for digestion.

This combination produces acid juices and alkaline juices at the same time. This combination produces water, which creates digestive juices that cannot fully digest either type of food.

In this case, the body produces more acid and more alkaline juices, which again are neutralized. The cycle continues until the food in your stomach starts to putrefy and ferment causing gas and acids. The gas causes belching and the combination gas and acids can lead to acid reflux.

As foods turn into acids because of the putrefaction and fermentation process, this food acid spoils all of the food in your stomach, causing undigested food to backflow up your esophagus and flow prematurely into your small intestine.

Food that is partially undigested becomes acidic, which affect the health of your colon, and when absorbed into your body is converted into fat and stored as a toxin in your body.

In many cases, the fermentation of food results in the production of alcohol and is similar to a person who drinks alcohol. There have been cases where people have been arrested for drunk driving and have never drank in their life and they wonder why they had a high blood alcohol level.

Eating the right combinations of foods at mealtime helps to preserve your energy for the elimination cycle and prevents you from creating spoiled food in your stomach that is converted to acid waste.

It is this acid waste that results in illness and fat. This is the reason most people as they age come down with various illnesses that terminate their life early or gain excessive weight.

14: Natural Body Cycle 3

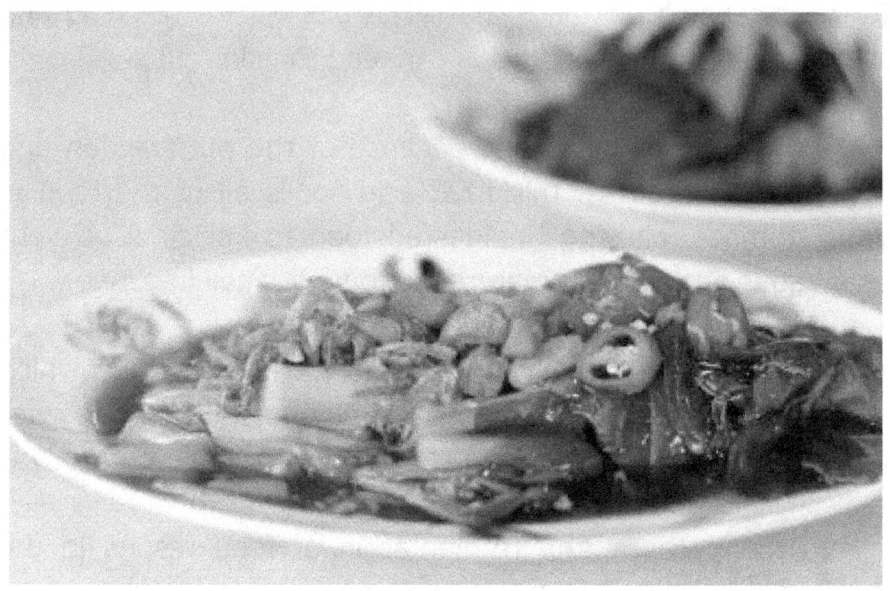

Cycle 3 is the assimilation cycle and is from 8 pm to 4 am. This is the time the food you have eaten during the day is assimilated, absorbed and distributed throughout your body through your blood.

Food that was eaten during cycle II and that was combined and eaten properly will digest within 3 hours. Whereas food that does not combine properly, a meal consisting of protein and carbohydrates will take up to 8 hours to pass through the stomach. During this time, your food will putrefy and ferment and become acidic. Under these conditions, you will not get any nutrients from that meal.

Natural Body Cycle 3

Eat your last meal by 6-7pm so that your food digests in your stomach by the time you go to bed. After three hours later, your food will have moved into your small intestine where it is ready for assimilation.

When you go to bed 3 hours after your last meal, the next 6 hours, until 4 am, your body will be absorbing the food you have eaten the previous day.

Remember, anything you do differently than what these cycles call for will disrupt them and cause them to become extended. When this happens, your food turns into acid, you don't absorb the value of your food, you lose energy and become tired, and over time you gain weight and create serious illnesses.

Have you ever notices how everyone you know eventually comes down with some sickness, which requires surgery or doctor's drugs. Think about it. Is this what you want happening to you? Just start changing your eating habits slowly and as time passes you will be doing more and more of what your body's natural cycles need.

15: Juice and Tonic Program

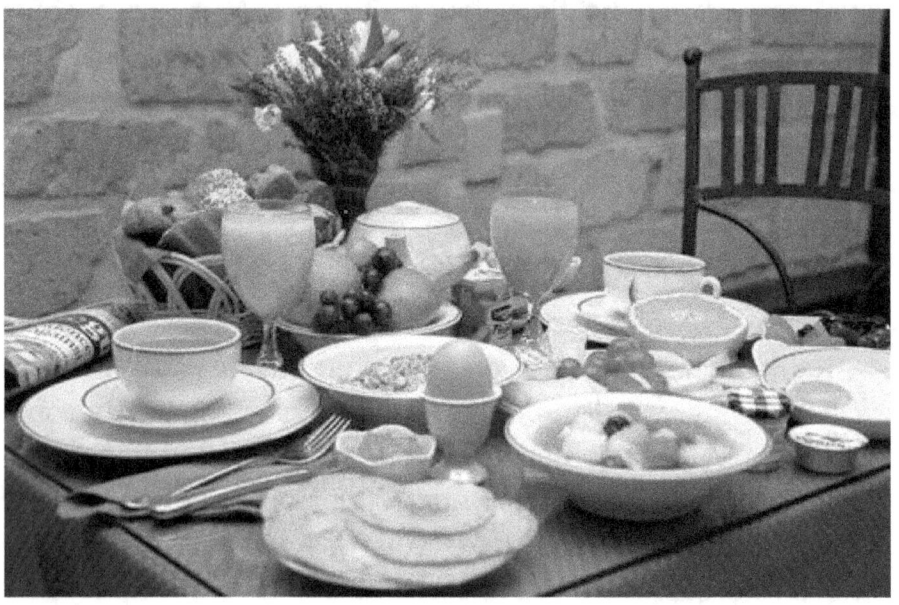

Ok there you have it, a large number of juices and tonics that you can use to accomplish whatever you want with your health and anti-aging program.

So, now where do you start with all this information? In this section, you will find one of the ways to use much of the information given to you in this book.

First of all, you need to re-familiarize yourself with the body cycles. You need to use these time periods to integrate the use of various juices and tonics during this cycle.

In cycle 1, from morning to noon time is when you will eat most of the fruits and juices and tonics.

In cycle 2 the only time that you have to use these drinks is during break time or about an hour before lunch and dinner.

In cycle 3 the only time here is to drink something before bedtime.

Cycle One Time Eating

When you first wake up, you want to drink any of the following:

1. Chose one of the tonics that will help you with a body condition you want to change. You can drink this anytime during the morning and afternoon.
2. If you want to drink your tonic later, then start with one of these drinks.
a. Warm or room temperature 8 oz. of water with the juice of one lemon
b. The chlorophyll drink with lemon and 8 oz. of water
c. A green drink powder
d. Green tea and ginger tea with honey.
e. Any fresh juice or combination of juices especially the citrus juices.
f. Any vegetable juice or combination that you want to use to target a specific condition.

The above drinks should be taken when you first get up and you can alternate with these drinks during the week or every week.

After your morning drink, wait about 30 to 45 minutes. You can now have your breakfast. This can consist of one of the following. If you want to eat oats, try to only have it once a week.

1. Fruit smoothie from the list provided – use leftovers for a midmorning snack.
2. A fruit pudding of a mixture of fruits in a blender with a little bit of juice.
3. A bowl of mixed fruits
4. A bowl of mixed melons and watermelon

For snacks, take some juice, smoothie, or tonic in a thermos for drinking before lunch or after lunch.

For lunch and dinner, re-read the section on body cycles and keep in tune with all the body cycles. Look over the tonics section and always be using a tonic with all your other drinks. Make sure you don't drink much with your lunch and dinner so that you can improve your digestion. Use digestive enzymes with each meal.

There you have it. There's plenty to do. Start now doing just a few things and build up your program over time.

16: The Author And Other Resources

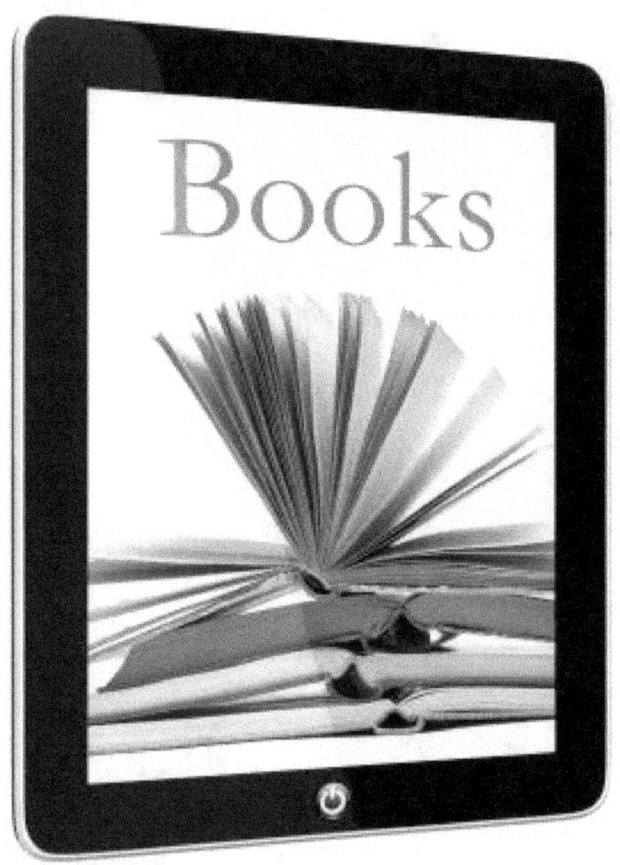

Rudy Silva is a natural consultant nutritionist educated in the United State of Nutrition and Physics.   He is a graduate of the San Jose State University in California. He is the author of 30 other e-books on natural remedies. He has authored a newsletter in natural remedies for over

4 years.　　He has many websites promoting special recommended products and information.

Resource page

Here are some of the other kindle e-books about natural remedies that have been written by this author.

1. Seven Day Colon and Blood Cleansing Diet – this e-book gives a step by step method of doing a colon and blood cleanse using fruits, vegetables, and their juices.

2.　Constipation Natural Cures – this is a comprehensive e-book on all aspects of constipation and colon health. In this e-book, you will find all the information you need on how your colon really works and what you need to do to get rid of constipation.

3. Acne Natural Treatments – This e-book outlines internal and external processes to use to stop the progression of facial acne. Natural remedies are given so that you can minimize the growth of pimples. You also are given a facial technique with various creams so that you can eliminate the external facial blemishes.

4. Hemorrhoid Natural Remedies - A variety of different remedies and techniques are outlined and given so that you can eliminate your hemorrhoids. Some remedies are provided from feedback given by clients.

5. Asthma Remedies – In this e-book, my daughter and I worked together to create a process that will help you minimize and even eliminated asthma using natural remedies. She has had asthma for many years and has discovered what diet she had to follow to prevent asthma attacks. This diet is provided with a variety of the most effective natural remedies that work on asthma and asthma attacks.

6. Essential Fatty Acids Explained – in this e-book, you will discover how essential fatty acids – omega-3 and omega-6 – work in your body. You will learn what diseases are created when you are deficient in essential fatty acids. Knowing this information will help you avoid these diseases and help you live a longer productive and pleasurable life.

7 Acid Reflux and Heartburn Diet – Gain a full understanding of what acid reflux is. Using this information, you will be able to see why the diet given really works. You will discover the natural remedies that you need to use to stabilize your stomach and to rejuvenate the tissue damage done in your stomach acid and in your esophagus.

If you need support or want to promote any of his e-books, please contact him at rss41@yahoo.com and expect a reply within 24 hours. He looks forward to hearing from you and is happy to help you understand his material on natural and nutritional health.

Give A Review

And, don't forget to give a review for this e-book so that others can gain the benefits of what is in this e-book.

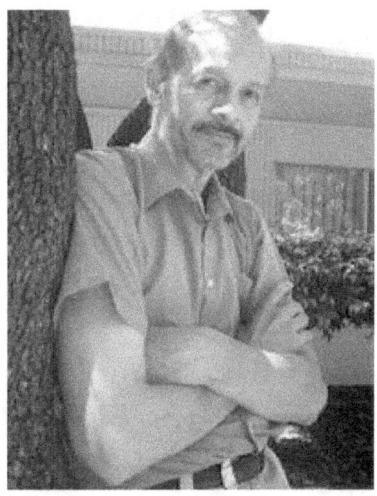

To you, for losing weight, creating better health and more happiness in your life,

Rudy S Silva

www.ingramcontent.com/pod-product-compliance
Lightning Source LLC
Chambersburg PA
CBHW070536290526
45790CB00002B/516